Basic Neuroscience for the Health Professions

Elizabeth H. Littell, PhD, PT

SLACK International Book Distributors

In Europe, The Middle East and Africa:
John Wiley & Sons Limited
Baffins Lane
Chichester, West Sussex PO19 1UD
England

In Canada
McAinsh and Company
2760 Old Leslie Street
Willowdale, Ontario M2K 2X5

In Australia and New Zealand:
MacLennan & Petty Pty Limited
P.O. Box 425
Artarmon, N.S.W. 2064
Australia

In Japan:
Igaku-Shoin, Ltd.
Tokyo International
P.O. Box 5063
1-28-36 Hongo, Bunkyo-Ku
Tokyo 113
Japan

In Asia and India:
PG Publishing Pte Limited.
36 West Coast Road, #02-02
Singapore 0512

Foreign Translation Agent
John Scott & Company
International Publishers' Agency
417-A Pickering Road
Phoenixville, PA 19460

Publisher: Harry C. Benson
Managing Editor: Lynn Borders
Editor: Cheryl D. Willoughby
Designer: Susan Hermansen
Production Manager: David Murphy

Printed in the United States of America

Library of Congress Catalog Card Number: 88-043482

ISBN: 1-55642-053-6

Published by: SLACK Incorporated
6900 Grove Rd.
Thorofare, NJ 08086

Last digit is print number: 10 9 8 7 6 5 4 3 2 1

for
Art and John

CONTENTS

LIST OF ILLUSTRATIONS

Chapter 4. Information Transfer

Chapter 5. Development, Degeneration, and
Regeneration in the Nervous System

Chapter 6. Spinal Cord Anatomy

Chapter 7. Spinal Sensorimotor Integration

Chapter 8. Brainstem Anatomy

Chapter 9. Brainstem Sensory Systems: Trigeminal, Gustatory, Cochlear, and Vestibular

LIST OF TABLES

PREFACE

Changes in scientific knowledge and in its application in the field of physical therapy have been impressive over the past 20 years. During this time there has been an explosion of knowledge in the discipline of neuroscience. Correspondingly, there have been significant changes in medical technology that have ensured the survival of many people with severe neurological problems. The role of physical therapy has been to integrate the expanding knowledge in neuroscience with the practice of therapy for persons with neurological problems. Treatment approaches such as those initiated in the years from the mid-1940s to the 1960s by therapists such as Margaret Knott and Dorothy Voss, Berta Bobath, Margaret Rood, Signe Brunnstrom, and Jean Ayers have been refined, modified, and, to a certain extent, integrated with each other. These exciting developments in treatment have imposed a responsibility on the physical therapy student to have a solid understanding of the basic structure and function of the nervous system as they enter practice.

This text is intended to provide a framework for understanding the nervous system and to give access to more advanced and detailed study in the area of applied neuroscience. The material included has been selected from the wide range of neuroscience information to fill the particular needs of the entry-level physical therapist. The emphasis in the text is on development of concepts of structure and function. This volume is not intended specifically as a doorway to research study; therefore, no attempt has been made to cite the extensive and continually growing neuroscience literature. The bibliographic list provides suggestions of texts that can be used to advance the study of current and historical research in neuroscience. The illustrations provided are to a large extent diagramatic and conceptual. The student will need access to a detailed atlas of the nervous system and to laboratory specimens and models to compliment the material presented in this volume. A list of atlases can be found in the bibliography.

I would like to acknowledge the help of the many students who have used this approach to an introduction to neuroscience over the past years. Their support and critical comments have had a considerable role in framing this presentation. I would also especially like to acknowledge the assistance of the illustrator of this volume, Steve Wright, who was willing to take on the challenge of learning enough neuroscience to translate my verbal concepts and rough sketches into reality.

E.H.L.

ABBREVIATIONS

Standard Scientific Notation

Å	Ångstrom
cm	centimeter
cm^3	cubic centimeter
gm	gram
Hz	Hertz or cycles per second
inf	inferior
L_o	resting length of a muscle
m	meter
min	minute
mg	milligram
ml	milliliter
mM	millimolar
mm	millimeter
mmHg	millimeters of mercury
msec	millisecond
mV	millivolt
μm	micron or micrometer
n. or nuc.	nucleus
$P_{(molecule)}$	partial pressure of the molecule
pH	logarithmic hydrogen concentration
sec	second
superscript "o" except in "primary" or "secondary": degree	
sup.	superior
1°	primary
2°	secondary

Abbreviations Introduced in Text, with Definitions

ACh	acetylcholine
AP	action potential
ARAS	ascending reticular activating system
B	basket cell
CNS	central nervous system
CSF	cerebrospinal fluid
CT	computerized tomography
EEG	electroencephalogram
FRA	flexor reflex afferent
GABA	gamma-amino butyric acid
GSA	general somatic afferent
GSE	general somatic efferent
GTO	Golgi tendon organ
GVA	general visceral afferent
GVE	general visceral efferent
MRI	magnetic resonance imaging
NMR	nuclear magnetic resonance
PAD	primary afferent depolarization
PAG	periaqueductal grey
PAH	primary afferent hyperpolarization
PET	positron emission tomography
PNS	peripheral nervous system
REM	rapid eye movement sleep
S_c	climbing stellate cell
S_h	horizontal stellate cell
SEP	sensory evoked potential
SSA	special somatic afferent
SVA	special visceral afferent
SVE	special visceral efferent
SWS	slow wave sleep
VA	ventral anterior nucleus
VL	ventral lateral nucleus
VPL	ventral posterior lateral nucleus
VPM	ventral posterior medial nucleus
5-HT	5 hydroxytryptamine
C1-C8, T1-T12, L1-L5, S1-S5, Coc1:	
	cervical, thoracic, lumbar, sacral and coccygeal spinal cord or vertebral levels, respectively

Gross Organization of the Nervous System

The nervous system consists of all neural cell bodies and their extensions, or processes, and cells that have functional supportive contact with neural cells. The main structural components of the nervous system in order from the most anterior portion are the cerebral hemispheres made up of cortex and basal ganglia; the diencephalon; the brainstem including the midbrain, pons, and medulla; the cerebellum; the spinal cord; the peripheral nerves including spinal nerves connected to the spinal cord and cranial nerves connected to the brainstem, diencephalon, or cerebral cortex; the autonomic ganglia; and the myenteric plexus of the gastrointestinal system (Fig. 1-1). Of these components, the peripheral nerves, the autonomic ganglia, and the myenteric plexus makeup the *peripheral nervous system* (PNS), and the remainder form the *central nervous system* (CNS). The division between these two major continuous parts of the nervous system is usually grossly obvious, but at the tissue level can only be made by examining the supporting rather than the neural cells. The supporting cells of one division are excluded completely from the other; however, in many cases neurons have cell bodies in one of the major divisions of the nervous system but have processes that extend into the other part.

Another frequently used division of the nervous system separates neurons into *autonomic* and *somatic* neurons. Somatic neurons control skeletal striated muscle; autonomic neurons provide more or less direct control of all other tissues in the body.

One of the major anatomical organizing principles of the CNS is that it developed as a bilaterally symmetrical tissue surrounding a central tube. The central tube develops into the adult ventricular system (Fig. 1-2). The central tube, or canal, is barely evident in the adult spinal cord. In the brainstem, there is an enlargement of the tube, the fourth ventricle, underlying the cerebellum. The tube narrows again in the upper brainstem, forming the aqueduct of Sylvius, or cerebral aqueduct. Another enlargement, the third

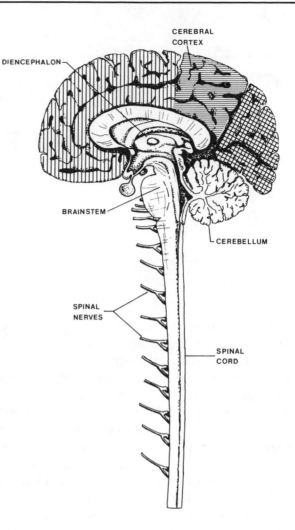

Figure 1-1. Mid-sagittal section of the central nervous system.

ventricle, is centered in the diencephalon. Because of the great growth of the cerebral hemispheres during development, the most anterior portion of the central tube divides into two major enlargements lying within the hemispheres. These lateral, or first and second ventricles, are connected with the third ventricle through the foramina of Munro. The ventricular system is filled with a specialized transcellular fluid, the cerebrospinal fluid, which is produced at secretory epithelium of the choroid plexi, located within the ventricles.

Another major organizing principle of the CNS is that there is extensive communication between the two sides of the system, with the result that many functional pathways project across the midline through bundles of neuron processes called *commissures*. Within the spinal cord ,there is a continuous anterior white commissure. In the brainstem, there is an extensive pattern of commissural crossings of various central tracts. The posterior-ventral region of the diencephalon contains additional subcortical commissures. The cere-

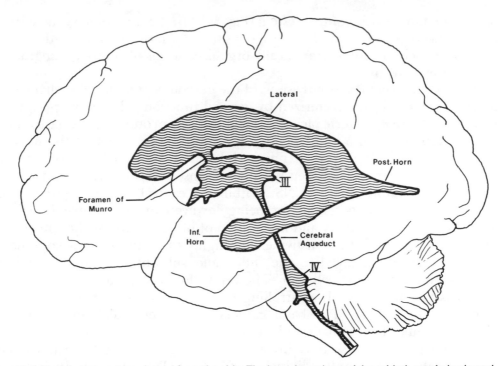

Figure 1-2. Ventricular system viewed from the side. The large lateral ventricles with the main body and posterior and inferior horns, are paired, one lying in each cerebral hemisphere. The two foramina of Munro connect the lateral ventricles to the third ventricle. All other ventricular spaces are unpaired, lying in the midline.

bral hemispheres have a number of commissural connections, the most noticeable among them being the corpus callosum connecting the cerebral cortex of both hemispheres and the anterior commissure connecting portions of the temporal lobe of the cerebral hemispheres and the limbic system. The latter is a phylogenetically old and anatomically dispersed functional subdivision of the cerebrum.

To function as a control system for the body as a whole, the nervous system must receive information, analyze it, and produce commands that will regulate the function of other tissues and organs. Functionally, neurons can be organized into those that receive information (*sensory*, often called afferent, neurons), those that organize information (*integration* or *association* neurons), and those that transmit commands (*motor*, often called efferent, neurons). These three basic functional types of neurons are found throughout the nervous system. In the PNS, integration neurons are found only in the autonomic ganglia and plexi and the myenteric plexus. In the CNS, the three types of neurons are found in every major anatomical subdivision, but they are distributed in very specific patterns. The study of neuroanatomy is concerned primarily with identifying these specific organizational distributions of types of neurons. At the simplest level, these three types of neurons can be organized into a basic control system (Fig. 1-3). In the human nervous system, most functions are carried out by considerably more complicated control systems, which include hierarchically organized levels of sensory, integration, and motor neurons.

The major structural subdivisions of the nervous system listed earlier can to a certain extent be characterized by general functions. The most peripheral component, the myenteric plexus, is responsible for control of the gastrointestinal system and can act independently from the remainder of the nervous system if disconnected from it. The peripheral nerves function as the sensory and motor connection between peripheral sensors and effectors and control centers (integrators) in the CNS. Within the central nervous system, each subdivision has the potential for being involved in all possible functions: sensory and motor activity and integration of information. At the spinal cord and brainstem level, these activities are highly programmed and automatic. These levels are involved in the reflex and subconscious control of both somatic and autonomic behavior. The cerebellum also is involved in subconscious behavior, primarily controlling the integration of somatic and autonomic motor activity. The basal ganglia of the cerebral hemispheres are involved primarily in somatic and autonomic motor control, but, in the human and other primates, also have involvement in higher cortical functions. The diencephalon is a complex division of the CNS. Part of it, the thalamus, is involved predominantly in regulating the delivery of all types of information to the cerebral cortex. Another part, the hypothalamus, is involved closely with integration and direction of autonomic function. The cerebral cortex serves as a terminal for sensory information of all types and as the originator

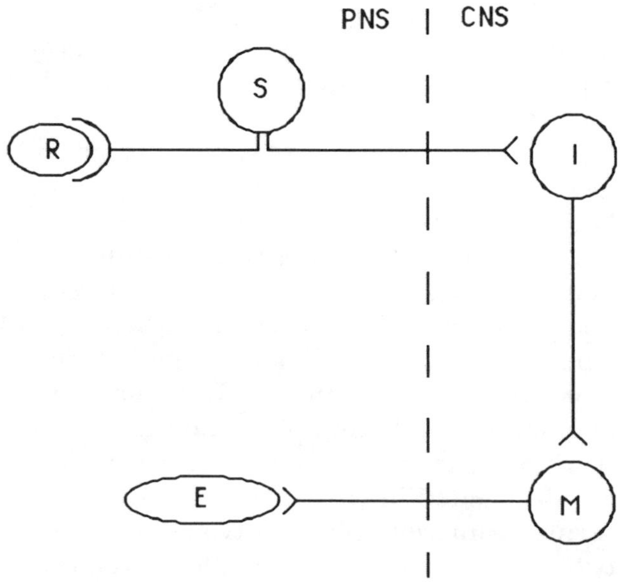

Figure 1-3. Elements of a simple neural system. *CNS,* central nervous system; *E,* peripheral effector tissue; *I,* integrator or association neuron; *M,* motor neuron; *PNS,* peripheral nervous system; *R,* sensory receptor; *S,* sensory neuron.

of voluntary somatic activity. It also is the center for very complex integrative functions that lead to the development of conscious behaviors of all kinds.

The cerebral hemispheres provide primarily complex integration functions. Sensory information of all types is received and integrated and elaborated into conscious sensory perception. Other conscious behaviors, such as language, various types of thinking and emotion, and memory, also have their anatomical substrate in the cerebrum. The main anatomical subdivisions, or lobes, of the cerebral hemispheres are the frontal, parietal, occipital, and temporal lobes (Fig. 1-4). Very generally speaking, motor function is located in the frontal lobe; sensory function in the parietal, occipital, and temporal lobes; and higher cortical functions in all lobes.

In the description of locations of structures in the central nervous system, standard anatomical planes of section are used with some modifications (Fig. 1-5). Anatomical sections of the cerebral hemispheres are made typically in the midsaggital and parasaggital planes, the coronal or vertical plane, and the horizontal plane. The diencephalon and brainstem are pictured typically in cross section perpendicular to the plane of the long axis of the central nervous system. Because of the nearly 90° flexion of the longitudinal axis between the cerebral hemispheres and the spinal cord, these diencephalic and brainstem cross sections are not continuously parallel to each other. Diencephalic cross sections are nearly in the coronal plane, and lower brainstem cross sections are nearly in the horizontal plane. These regions of the CNS may also be viewed in longitudinal section, which is nearly parallel to a coronal section of the

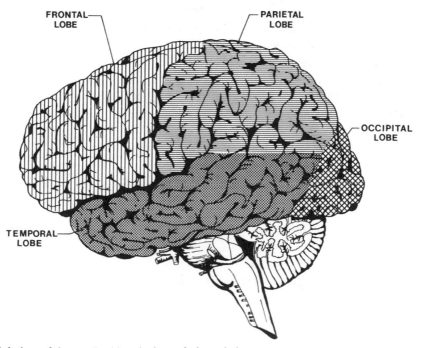

Figure 1-4. Lobes of the cerebral hemispheres in lateral view.

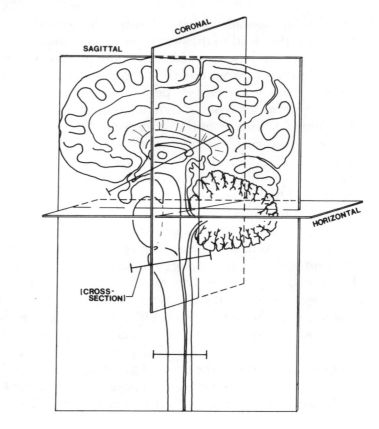

Figure 1-5. Midsagittal view of the central nervous system showing standard planes of section. Note the change in angulation of cross-sections from the diencephalon to the spinal cord.

cerebral hemispheres. The cerebellum is shown either in parasaggital section or cross section paralleling cross sections of the adjacent brainstem. The internal spinal cord is represented typically in cross sections, which are in the horizontal plane. Additional planes of section may be used either in specialized anatomical studies or in clinical imaging. Whenever unusual planes of section are being used, the angle of the plane with the horizontal is indicated.

Coverings of the Nervous System

The entire central nervous system is enclosed within a triple layer of protective connective tissue, the meninges, with each layer having its own special function (Fig. 1-6).

The outermost layer, the dura mater, is a thick, tough fibrous connective tissue membrane with minimal elasticity. It surrounds the meningeal arteries

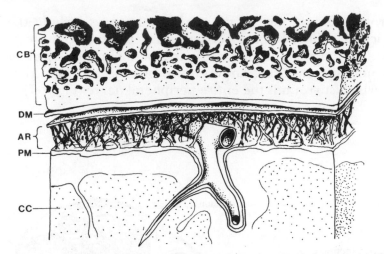

Figure 1-6. Meningeal layers of the central nervous system as seen overlying the cerebral hemispheres. *AR,* arachnoid with trabeculae bridging the subarachnoid space; *CB,* cortical bone; *CC,* cerebral cortex; *DM,* dura mater; *PM,* pia mater. An artery is shown passing through the subarachnoid space and penetrating the hemisphere.

and veins and the major veins draining the CNS proper. The outer layer of the dura is adherent to the skull but separated from the vertebral bodies by a cushioning layer of fatty tissue. At the lower end of the spinal canal, the dura is attached to the coccyx, forming the filum terminale and the coccygeal ligament. The dura extends out from the CNS a short distance along the peripheral nerves and dips into the CNS in two major cortical fissures inside the skull. These major extensions of the dura are the falx cerebri, which descends in the dorsal longitudinal fissure down to the level of the corpus callosum and thus separates the two cerebral hemispheres, and the tentorium cerebelli, which lies horizontally between the dorsum of the cerebellum and the ventral surface of the posterior cerebral hemispheres.

The middle meningeal layer, the arachnoid, is formed of a fine filamentous network bridging the fluid-filled subarachnoid space between the dura and the inner meningeal layer. Cerebrospinal fluid circulates in this space, providing a hydraulic cushion for the CNS. Blood vessels entering and leaving the substance of the CNS run through the arachnoid.

The innermost layer, the pia mater, is a continuous, single-thickness layer adherent to the surface of the CNS. It runs with arteries and veins a variable distance into the CNS and participates to a certain extent in the blood-brain barrier of the central nervous system.

The protective coverings of the peripheral nerves include the endoneurium, which is a fine, single-layer covering enclosing one or a few nerve processes and their supporting cells; the perineurium, which is a slightly thicker membrane enclosing large groups of processes; and the tough epineurium, which surrounds the entire peripheral nerve (Fig. 1-7).

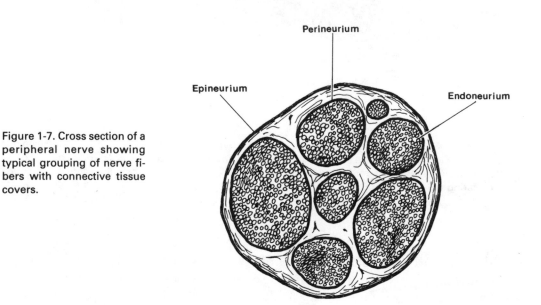

Figure 1-7. Cross section of a peripheral nerve showing typical grouping of nerve fibers with connective tissue covers.

Review Exercises

1-1.   Four patients are described in the Appendix. For each of these patients, identify on Figures 1-1 and 1-4 the general location of the lesion(s) causing their problem.

1-2.   Classify the neurons listed below on the basis of their primary character or function as you currently understand it, using as classification categories the following: 1) autonomic neuron, 2) somatic neuron, 3) sensory neuron, 4) motor neuron, 5) association or integration neuron, 6) myenteric neuron. Use more than one classification when appropriate.
    a. neuron involved in remembering information
    b. neuron controlling excitation of the biceps brachii
    c. neuron controlling intestinal peristalsis
    d. neuron carrying pain information from the big toe
    e. neuron regulating heart rate
    f. neuron receiving information concerning both blood pressure and blood gas concentration

1-3.   If the aqueduct of Sylvius is obstructed and the choroid plexi of the two lateral ventricles and the midline third ventricle continue to produce cerebrospinal fluid, describe what you would expect to have happen to the tissues listed below. Justify your answers.

a. dura matter covering the cerebral hemispheres
b. the spinal cord
c. the brainstem
d. veins and arteries in the subarachnoid space
e. the cerebellum
f. the diencephalon
g. the cerebral hemispheres

2

Histology and Cytoarchitecture of the Nervous System

The nervous system contains three basic types of cells: neurons, supporting cells, and protecting cells. Neurons provide for information transfer and storage. Supporting cells provide metabolic, structural, biophysical, and immunological support for neurons. Protecting cells, described earlier as the meninges and the connective tissue sheaths of peripheral nerves, provide mechanical support and protection for neural and associated circulatory structures.

Neurons

All neurons, regardless of specific function, share basic structural characteristics (Fig. 2-1). Neurons have two major functional and anatomical divisions: the cell body and the neuron processes branching from the cell body to make functional contact with other neurons or effector cells. Neurons have specialized communication regions, the presynaptic and postsynaptic regions. Presynaptic regions are located on processes, and postsynaptic regions are found on both processes and the cell body itself. The bulk of the manufacturing equipment of the cell, such the nucleus, endoplasmic reticulum, and Golgi apparatus, is located in the cell body. As in most cells, the endoplasmic reticulum has both smooth and rough sections. The rough endoplasmic reticulum of neurons is particularly susceptible to staining by certain types of histological stains, the first of which were developed by Nissl. For this reason, the endoplasmic reticulum of neurons frequently is referred to as Nissl substance. Synapses contain vesicles that also have circumscribed manufacturing capability. Mitochondria, which supply energy, are located in the cell body, within processes where electrochemical activity is pronounced, and at synap-

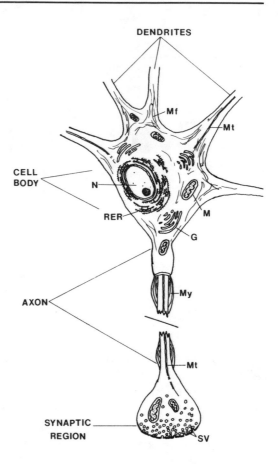

Figure 2-1. Components of a typical neuron. *G,* Golgi material; *M,* mitochondrion; *My,* myelin sheath; *N,* nucleus; *Mf,* microfilament; *Mt,* microtubule; *RER,* rough endoplasmic reticulum (Nissl substance); *SV,* synaptic vesicles.

ses. Transport structures, which are the microtubules and microfilaments of the neuronal processes, support movement of cellular chemicals between the cell body and process terminals. Storage vesicles containing neurotransmitters are found predominantly in the presynaptic regions of processes.

Transport of cellular material or electrical impulses away from the cell body is termed *efferent* transport. Transport toward the cell body is termed *afferent.* Cell processes are named on the basis of the predominant direction of movement of electrical impulses within them. Thus, axons predominantly conduct electrical impulses away from the cell body, and dendrites conduct them toward the cell. There are, however, numerous exceptions to this rule; dendrites in particular are involved in both afferent and efferent impulse conduction.

Neurons are characterized on the basis of cell body size and the number and branching pattern of their processes (Fig. 2-2). Neurons with only one process capable of bidirectional impulse transmission are termed *unipolar.* The human nervous system contains no such neurons. *Bipolar* and *pseudounipolar* neurons have one afferent and one efferent process connected to the cell body. In pseudounipolar neurons, the two processes are immediately adjacent to each other close to the cell body and appear grossly to be a single process.

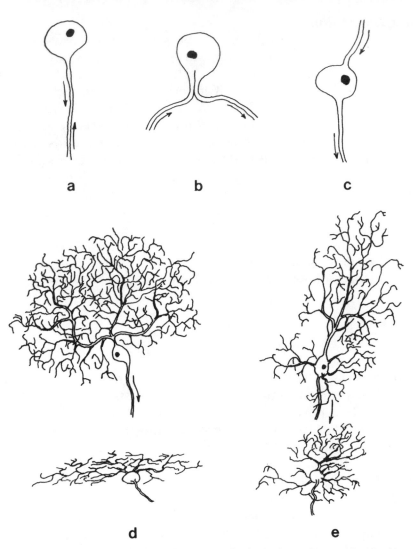

Figure 2-2. Neuron process branching patterns. **a.** unipolar neuron; **b.** pseudounipolar neuron; **c.** bipolar neuron; **d.** and **e.** multipolar neurons. **d** represents a cerebellar cortex Purkinje cell with its typical single plane fan-like dendritic tree. **e** represents a cerebral cortex pyramidal neuron with apical and basal dendrites branching in all planes from the cell body.

All other neurons are *multipolar*. The pattern of process branching is not random for any cell but is defined specifically by genetic and trophic factors during development. Some neurons have no morphologically identifiable axon, but they use dendrites for both afferent and efferent exchange of information. The size of neurons is extremely variable. Cell body diameter ranges from 6 μm to 100 μm, and the process diameter ranges from 0.1 μm to 20 μm. The length of individual processes varies from less than 1 μm to about 1 m, a range of 6 orders of magnitude. Cell body shape also is varied and characteristic for certain types of neurons.

Histological Stains

Different cellular components can be stained using various histological stains. The staining properties of the various cells in the CNS must be understood to interpret sections correctly. The cell body of neurons is stained discretely by Nissl type stains, which adhere selectively to the rough endoplasmic reticulum. Nissl stains will color neuron cell bodies, leaving neuron processes and myelin unstained. Glial cell bodies stain variably with Nissl stains. Neuron cell membranes stain selectively with Golgi-type stains. Such stains are used to demonstrate the cell body and processes of neurons and are useful when identifying individual neurons in serial sections. Golgi stains tend to be selective, staining only a small percentage of the neurons in any given section; however, any neuron stained is stained in its entirety. Myelin or Weigart-type stains preferentially color myelin, thereby giving definition to fiber pathways, most of which in the CNS are myelinated to at least some degree. Gross anatomical sections of the CNS are prepared typically either with Nissl stains for cell body definition, which is useful when studying the detailed cytoarchitecture of collections of cell bodies, or with myelin stains for fiber pathway definition.

Supporting Cells

The supporting cells of the nervous system are not involved directly in the transfer of information but supply metabolic, structural, biophysical, and immunological support to neurons. Within the CNS, support cells are termed *glia* (Fig. 2-3). They can be broken down into the following structural and functional subclasses:

1. Oligodendroglia (oligodendrocytes, oligoglia): form myelin sheaths around axons within the CNS, thus providing biophysical, structural, and possibly some metabolic support.
2. Astroglia (astrocytes): form an anatomical bridge between neurons and CNS capillaries; their function probably is metabolic support, including buffering of changes in extracellular ionic concentration. They may act also as phagocytes. There are two morphological types of astroglia: fibrous and protoplasmic.
3. Microglia: small mobile and proliferative cells that provide phagocytosis in cases of trauma or infection.
4. Ependyma: cuboidal cells, lining the ventricular system, that participate in fluid transport within the CNS. A specialized type of ependymal cell is found in the choroid epithelium of the ventricles.

The supporting cells of the PNS include the Schwann cells, which myelinate neuronal processes in peripheral nerves (Figs. 2-4, 2-5), and the capsule cells of the PNS ganglia (collections of nerve cell bodies). The Schwann cells provide biophysical, metabolic and immunological support functions; the function of the capsule cells is probably similar.

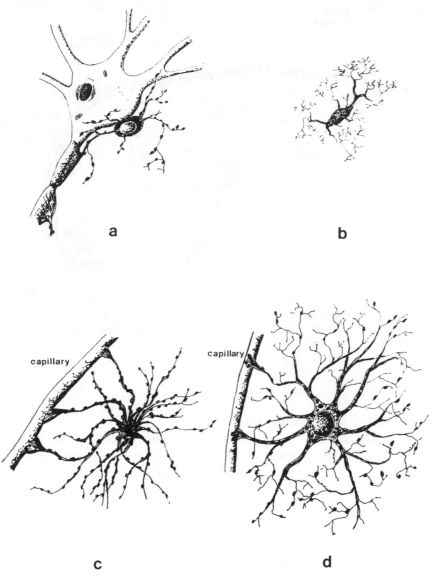

Figure 2-3. Central nervous system glial cells. **a.** oligodendroglia with processes forming the myelin sheath around an axon; **b.** microglia; **c.** protoplasmic astrocyte; **d.** fibrous astrocyte. The processes of both types of astrocyte come into close proximity to capillary endothelium.

Cytoarchitecture

Cytoarchitecture refers to the typical arrangement of nerve cell bodies (grey matter) and processes (white matter) within the nervous system. In all parts of the nervous system, the arrangement of cell bodies and processes is highly specific and closely related to function.

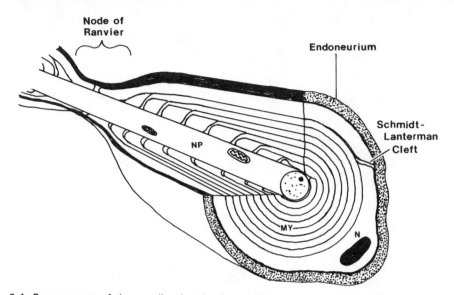

Figure 2-4. Components of the myelin sheath of a peripheral nerve process. *MY,* layers of myelin formed by the specialized cell membrane of the Schwann cell; *N,* Schwann cell neuron; *NP,* neuron process. The layers of myelin end at the node of Ranvier. The boundary of the spiral wrapping of myelin occurs at the Schmidt-Lanterman cleft. The endoneurial connective tissue is closely applied to the outside of the Schwann cell.

Central Neural Cytoarchitecture

There are three basic structural arrangements of cell bodies (grey matter) within the CNS: deep nuclear groups, surface layers, and diffuse deep networks. Cells in deep nuclei and in cortical layers usually show very specific layered or clustered organization that is correlated strongly with specific cell

Figure 2-5. Cross section of peripheral nerve fibers. **a** Myelinated fiber; **b** Unmyelinated fiber enclosed in a Schwann cell but lacking the myelin wrappings of the cell membrane. Frequently more than one unmyelinated fiber will be enclosed in one Schwann cell. *MY,* myelin sheath; *N,* nucleus of Schwann cell; *NP,* neuron process or fiber.

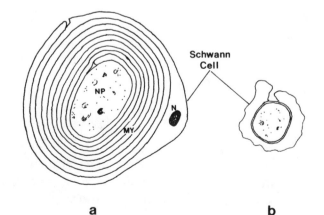

a   b

morphology and function. Cortical layers frequently are folded extensively, as in the cerebrum and the cerebellum, which increases the available surface area into which cells can be placed. Cellular networks are organized more openly (at least to the eye) and are composed of large numbers of similar cells in more or less compact aggregations and interconnected with each other in multiple ways. A prime example of a network is the reticular formation found in the brainstem.

Neuronal processes entering or leaving cellular areas tend to be grouped into fiber bundles (tracts or pathways) on the basis of their origin, destination, and common function. Fiber bundles form the white matter of the CNS (so-called because of the relatively light color of myelin in fresh material). Fiber bundles are made up of processes of varying diameter, with greater and lesser degrees of myelination. In the cerebral and cerebellar cortex, the white matter is deep to the cortical cellular layers; in the brainstem, fiber bundles are to a certain extent intermingled with cellular regions; and in the spinal cord, the long fiber pathways are external to the layered central grey matter. Long fiber bundles can serve as useful landmarks through the CNS.

The cerebral and cerebellar hemispheres have a basically similar cytoarchitecture. Both have outer cortical layers separated from groups of deep nuclei by a layer of fibers (Figs. 2-6, 2-7). These fibers serve to connect the cortical

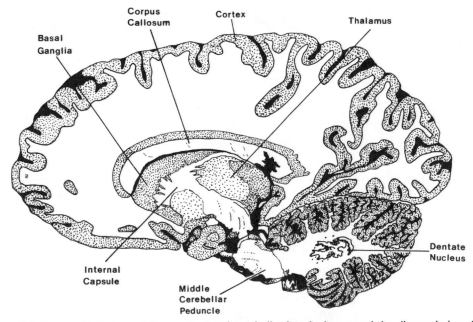

Figure 2-6. Parasagittal view of the cerebral and cerebellar hemispheres and the diencephalon. Cell body regions are stippled. The cortical layers of both the cerebrum and the cerebellum overlie the white matter fiber pathways. Contained deep within the white matter of the cerebrum and cerebellum are the deep nuclei (basal ganglia and dentate nucleus). The thalamus forms a region of nuclei within the diencephalon. The internal capsule is a major fiber pathway within the diencephalon.

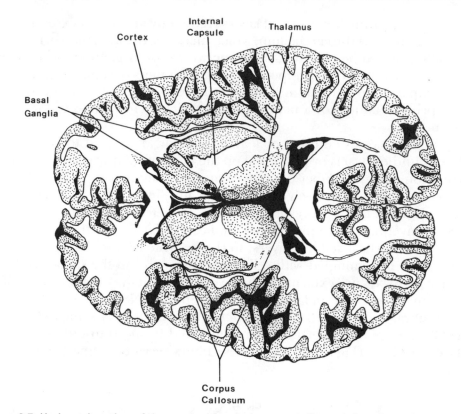

Figure 2-7. Horizontal section of the cerebral hemispheres and diencephalon above the plane of the cerebellum.

layers with structures outside the cerebellum or cerebrum and to provide interconnections among cortical regions and between the cortex and the deep nuclei. The deep nuclei (basal ganglia in the cerebral hemispheres, deep or roof nuclei in the cerebellum) are composed of highly organized clusters of cell bodies.

The diencephalon predominantly contains nuclei segregated on a functional basis. Some diencephalic nuclei contain cells organized in clusters, but others show a distinct laminar organization. Major fiber pathways also occur within the diencephalon, with the most noticeable being the internal capsule containing fibers connecting the cerebral hemispheres with the diencephalon and lower CNS structures.

The brainstem is made up of a mixture of long fiber pathways, well-organized nuclei (with cells in clusters or laminae), and a network of cells, which is the brainstem reticular formation (Fig. 2-8). Most of the nuclei are related directly either to cranial nerves or to motor control pathways.

The spinal cord has the simplest cytoarchitecture of any of the subdivisions of the CNS. A central nuclear region with clear laminar organization is surrounded by fiber pathways (Fig. 2-9).

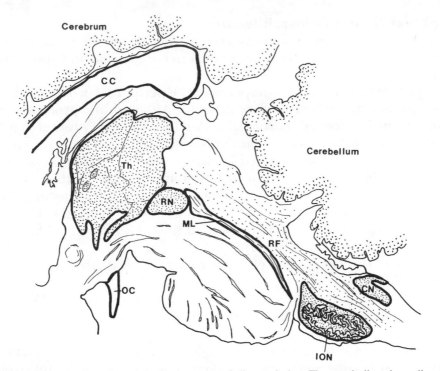

Figure 2-8. Parasagittal section of the brainstem and diencephalon. The cerebellum is outlined in the upper right, and part of the cerebral hemisphere in the upper left. *CC,* corpus collosum. A major fiber pathway connecting the right and left cerebral hemispheres; *CN,* cuneate nucleus of the medulla; *ION,* inferior olivary nucleus of the medulla; *MLF,* medial longitudinal fasciculus, a major fiber tract running the length of the brainstem; *OC,* optic chiasm; *RF,* reticular formation in the pons; *RN,* red nucleus of the midbrain.

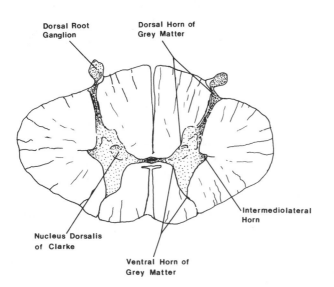

Figure 2-9. Cross section of the thoracic spinal cord. The dorsal root ganglia contain the cell bodies of sensory neurons.

Peripheral Neural Cytoarchitecture

The major structures to be considered in the PNS are the peripheral nerves proper, the spinal dorsal root and cranial nerve ganglia, and the autonomic ganglia.

The peripheral nerves are composed of the peripheral processes of somatic and autonomic motor and sensory neurons. Although the processes are to a certain extent intermixed, particularly distally, there is a predominant localization of fibers within a nerve on the basis of origin, destination, and function. All processes are surrounded by Schwann cells. Peripheral processes of neurons have been categorized by different investigators on the basis of their diameter, degree of myelination, conduction velocity, and function. The currently used classification schemes are summarized in Table 2-1. On the basis of these classifications, one can expect to find the following fiber types in various kinds of peripheral nerves:

1. Nerve to skeletal muscle: efferent A and C fibers; afferent Ia, Ib, II, III and IV fibers.
2. Nerve to skin: efferent C fibers; afferent II (beta), III and IV fibers.
3. Nerve to internal organs: efferent B and C fibers; afferent III and IV fibers.

Spinal dorsal root and cranial nerve ganglia contain the rounded cell bodies of the pseudounipolar sensory neurons; their processes, which are unmyelinated close to the cell body; and small supporting capsular cells. The dorsal roots themselves contain only sensory neuron processes. The ventral roots of spinal nerves contain both motor and sensory neuron processes in varying percentages (up to 30% sensory). The sensory fibers found in the ventral roots are primarily of group III and IV (Fig. 2-10). The cell bodies for these ventral fibers appear to be located in the dorsal root ganglia. The central processes retrace their route back to the junction of dorsal and ventral roots to enter the spinal cord through the ventral root. Collateral branches of these central processes may enter the spinal cord through the dorsal root.

Peripheral nerves are connected to one of the following sections of the CNS:

1. Spinal cord (spinal nerves).
2. Brainstem (cranial nerves III - XII).
3. Diencephalon (cranial nerve II).
4. Cerebral hemispheres (cranial nerve I).

Cranial nerves are not organized as uniformly as spinal nerves. The structure and functional components of the cranial nerves will be discussed in those chapters dealing with the brainstem (Chap. 8 and 9), the visual system (Chap. 17) and the limbic system (Chap. 18).

Autonomic ganglia are encapsulated structures similar in structure to dorsal root ganglia, but they also contain small interneurons and the cell bodies of peripheral autonomic neurons. Capsule cells also are found in autonomic ganglia. Fibers originating in, ending in, and passing through the autonomic ganglia include the following (Fig. 2-11):

TABLE 2-1. Categorization of Peripheral Nerve Processes

Class	Type	Group	Subgroup	Diameter (μm)	Conduction Velocity (m/sec)	Peripheral Contact
Sensory (afferent)						
Myelinated	A	I	Ia	12-20	72-120	muscle spindle 1°
			Ib	12-20	72-120	Golgi tendon organ
		II		6-12	36-72	muscle spindle 2°
		II (beta)		6-12	36-72	· skin pressure sensors · skin fine touch sensors
		III(delta)		1-6	6-36	· soft tissue pressure sensors · muscle and soft tissue pain sensors · skin gross touch sensors · skin temperature sensors · skin pain sensors
Unmyelinated	C	IV		~1	0.5-2	· muscle and soft tissue pain sensors · skin gross touch sensors · skin temperature sensors · skin pain sensors
Motor (efferent)						
Myelinated	A	alpha		12-20	72-120	skeletal striated muscle (extrafusal fibers)
		beta		10-15	50-100	skeletal striated muscle (extrafusal and intrafusal fibers)
		gamma		2-8	12-48	skeletal striated muscle (intrafusal fibers)
	B	preganglionic autonomic		~3	3-15	· postganglionic autonomic neurons · adrenal medulla
Unmyelinated	C	postganglionic autonomic		~1	0.5-2	· smooth muscle · glands · adipocytes

1. Preganglionic autonomic motor fibers (type B) reaching the ganglion through the white ramus from the spinal nerve root and terminating in the ganglion on postganglionic cells.
2. Postganglionic autonomic motor fibers (type C) originating in the ganglion and leaving the ganglion to join the peripheral nerve by way of the grey ramus.
3. Sensory fibers relating to the autonomic system, which may enter the ganglion through either ramus and split off collateral branches within the ganglion before continuing on to the spinal cord.

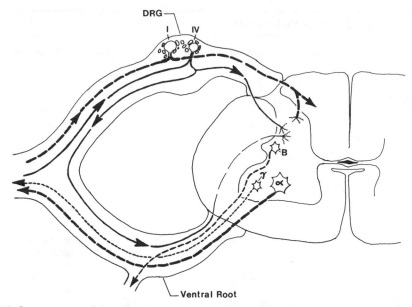

Figure 2-10. Components of dorsal and ventral roots of a typical spinal nerve. Large myelinated fibers (eg. group I) have cell bodies in the dorsal root ganglion. Their central processes enter the spinal cord and either synapse in the dorsal horn or ascend in the spinal white matter. Small unmyelinated fibers (eg. group IV) also have cell bodies in the dorsal root ganglion. Their central processes enter the dorsal horn and typically synapse there. Collateral branches of the central processes may pass back through the dorsal root and turn to enter the cord through the ventral root. Efferent, motor fibers in the ventral root arise from gamma (γ) and alpha (α) somatomotor neurons and Type B autonomic preganglionic neurons.

Synaptic Structure

A variety of possible junctions exists between neurons (Fig. 2-12). Several of these, including juxtapositions, desmosomes, and gap junctions, are found also in other tissue. A juxtaposition may permit some interchange of molecules, and may also permit exchange of electrical charge (in both directions), in which case the juxtaposition is termed an ephapse. Desmosomes are also termed tight junctions, septate junctions, or zonulae adherens. They may provide for exchange of material between adjacent cells, and they usually limit the movement of extracellular fluid past cells. Gap junctions are specialized desmosomes of small diameter with a 20 to 40 Å intracellular space. There is continuity of cytoplasm through the membrane pores between adjacent cells. Gap junctions provide for either unidirectional or bidirectional transfer of information through ion movement between connected cells. In the CNS, gap junctions are found among other places in several brainstem nuclei: the mesencephalic (midbrain) nucleus of the trigeminal nerve, Deiter's (vestibular) nucleus in the pons, and the inferior olive of the medulla.

Synapses are specialized junctions found only between neurons or between neurons and effector cells. All synapses share the characteristic of providing for information transfer between cells by the release of specific chemicals

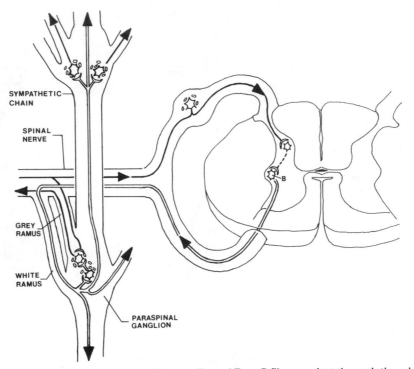

Figure 2-11. Autonomic spinal neurons. The myelinated Type B fibers project through the white ramus into the paraspinal autonomic ganglia of the sympathetic system. They may synapse in the first ganglion reached, pass through the ganglion to project to prespinal ganglia or plexi, or pass through the ganglion to project in the sympathetic chain to other paraspinal ganglia before synapsing. Postganglionic Type C fibers leave the ganglia through the grey ramus to rejoin the common spinal nerve. Interneurons may be positioned between B fibers and postganglionic neurons within the ganglia. Sensory afferents may connect with Type B cells within the spinal cord or may send collaterals to synapse directly with postganglionic neurons in the ganglia.

from the presynaptic cell and their uptake by specific receptors on the postsynaptic cell. Any given individual synapse is unidirectional, but bidirectional communication among neurons can occur easily at adjacent synapses connecting the same two cells. Furthermore, at some synapses, the released chemical can act on both the presynaptic and the postsynaptic cell. A synapse is made up of a presynaptic region on one cell and a postsynaptic region on the adjacent cell, separated by the synaptic cleft. The presynaptic region contains the chemical(s) released during synaptic activity. In most neurons, these chemicals are packaged in vesicles. The vesicles are organized spatially within the presynaptic region by a grid arrangement that is integral to the cell membrane. The postsynaptic region has a specialized cell membrane that contains specific receptors for the synaptic chemicals. Both presynaptic and postsynaptic regions contain a high concentration of mitochondria to support the relatively high level of metabolic activity associated with synaptic function. The presynaptic and postsynaptic regions may have a specialized morphology or may be relatively undifferentiated regions on the neuron process. An

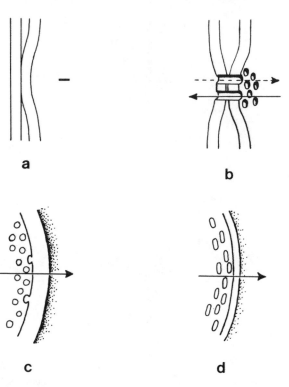

Figure 2-12. Neural junctions. **a** juxtaposition or ephapse showing a separation of charge between two adjacent cells. **b** gap junction showing routes for ion movement in one predominant direction. **c** Type I chemical synapse. **d** Type II chemical synapse.

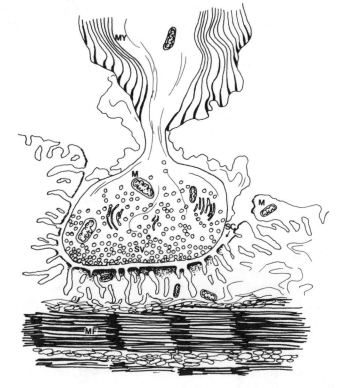

Figure 2-13. Neuromuscular junction. The axon terminal is unmyelinated and is embedded in the synaptic region of the striated muscle cell. Mitochondria are concentrated in both the pre- and postsynaptic regions to support the high level of metabolic activity associated with synaptic transmission. *M,* mitochondrion; *MF,* myofibrils; *MY,* myelin; *SC,* synaptic cleft; *SV,* synaptic vesicles containing neurotransmitter.

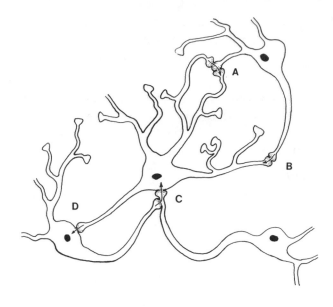

Figure 2-14. Typical central nervous system synapse locations. **A,** dendrodendritic synapse complex showing information transmission from the dendritic tree of one cell to the dendrite of another cell and back to the dendritic tree of the original cell. This type of a synapse permits a type of bidirectional synaptic activity and the presence of the intervening neuron dendrite allows for modification of the information. **B,** axo-dendritic synapse. **C,** complex showing an axo-somatic synapse accompanied by an axo-axonic synapse. **D,** simple axo-somatic synapse.

example of a morphologically complex synapse is the neuromuscular junction (Fig. 2-13). Synapse morphology is sufficiently distinctive that it can be used in identifying specific cell types. There are several different structural types of synapses and a number of possible synaptic arrangements between communicating cells. The basic morphological characteristics of the two primary types of synapses are outlined in Table 2-2. The anatomically more complex Type I synapses are typically excitatory in their effect on the postsynaptic cell; the Type II synapses are typically inhibitory. In addition to synapses on neuron processes, synapses frequently occur between the axon of a presynaptic cell and the soma of the postsynaptic cell (Fig. 2-14).

TABLE 2-2. Functional and Morphological Characteristics of Type I and Type II Chemical Synapses

Characteristics	Type I	Type II
Membrane Density	asymmetric	symmetric
Cleft Width	300 Å	200 Å
Vesicle Characteristics	spherical 300 - 600 Å diam. relatively sparse	ellipsoid 100 - 300 Å diam. abundant
Typical Postsynaptic Effect	excitation	inhibition

Review Exercises

2-1.   Identify all the locations in a typical neuron at which one would expect to find mitochondria. Justify your selection by discussing the type of energy requirements at each location.

2-2. Refer to Patient #2 in the Appendix. This patient has probably suffered injury to which of the types of peripheral nerve fibers described in this chapter? Justify your list on the basis of the type and location of structures you know to be innervated by the ulnar nerve.

2-3. Synapses are complex structures which require relatively large amounts of energy to function effectively. Consider what advantages there may be to basing an information processing system on such structures rather than on simpler and less energy-consumptive systems as ephapses or gap junctions.

2-4. Cell processes, both axons and dendrites, are found in both white and grey matter. What does the color distinction of these two types of neural tissue tell you about the types of glia found in each tissue and the degree of myelination of processes?

3

Anatomical Substrate for Sensation

Sensation is the process of receiving, transducing, and transmitting information about the current state of the external and internal environment of the body. Sensation does not require or include conscious awareness of stimuli, or perception, but it is a necessary prerequisite for normal perception. The characteristics of sensation that can be defined, described, and measured include the following:

1. Sensory modality: the "what" of sensation.
2. Sensation intensity: the "how much" of sensation.
3. Stimulus position: the "where" of sensation.
4. Stimulation timing: the "when" of sensation.

These parameters are determined in sensory systems by an interaction among sensory receptors, the pattern of activation of sensory neurons, and the location of neural synapses in the CNS.

The anatomical substrate for sensation is made up of three basic components: receptors; primary sensory neurons, or afferents,innervating the receptors; and higher order sensory reception and integration neurons. Receptors generally are identifiable, more or less differentiated, cells of ectodermal, mesodermal, or endodermal origin that bear a specific morphological relationship to the end of the peripheral process of a primary sensory neuron. Primary sensory neurons typically have a cell body outside of the CNS in a dorsal root or cranial nerve ganglion, a peripheral process extending in a peripheral nerve to the receptor, and a central process that enters the CNS to communicate with higher order sensory system neurons. There are some exceptions to this basic morphological picture: Cell bodies of neurons of the olfactory nerve (cranial nerve I) and part of the trigeminal nerve (mesencephalic nucleus of cranial nerve V) are located inside the CNS. Some sensory neurons, such as the osmoreceptors of the hypothalamus, are contained completely within the central nervous system, and some sensory neurons related to the autonomic system have peripheral processes that communicate with cells in autonomic ganglia or plexi. Sensory neurons that are contained wholly in the PNS may be found in the myenteric plexus. Higher order sensory neurons are located throughout the CNS and in the retina. Classically, it has been assumed that the peripheral processes of sensory neurons have only afferent function. Recent studies of pain function have indicated that at least the smaller afferent fibers (groups III and IV) can release neurotransmitters at their peripheral terminals, thus adding an efferent function.

Sensory receptors may be classified in terms of their modality, their morphology, the location of the stimuli to which they preferentially respond, and the response characteristics of their associated primary afferents. There are five types of receptors as classified by modality:

1. Mechanoreceptors: stimulated by mechanical deformation of the immediate tissue.
   Examples: Pacinian corpuscles, Meissner's corpuscles, Ruffini endings, hair follicle receptors, muscle spindles, Golgi tendon organs, cochlear hair cells, vestibular cells, free nerve endings, joint receptors.
2. Chemoreceptors: stimulated by specific chemicals or classes of chemicals in the immediate environment.
   Examples: olfactory neurons, taste bud receptors, free nerve endings, carotid body receptors, osmoreceptors.
3. Thermoreceptors: stimulated by changes in heat in the immediate environment.
   Examples: small encapsulated receptors, Krause end-bulbs, free nerve endings.
4. Nociceptors: stimulated by actually or potentially destructive mechanical, chemical or thermal changes in the immediate tissue
   Examples: small encapsulated receptors, free nerve endings.
5. Electromagnetic receptors: stimulated by electromagnetic radiation
   Examples: rods and cones of the retina.

A brief examination of this list indicates that the modality specificity of a receptor is not necessarily determined by its morphology; free nerve endings (which essentially do not have a receptor per se) are capable of receiving stimuli in a variety of modalities. The morphology and location within tissue of a given receptor do specify the modality received. The function of the morphology of the receptor capsule is to limit and direct ("focus") the type of energy that can stimulate the nerve ending. The response characteristics of a given receptor can be described by a "tuning curve" for the receptor (Fig. 3-1).

Morphologically, receptors fall into one of six possible categories:

1. Specialized sense organs: receptor cells and primary afferent terminals enclosed within an elaborate structure that serves to direct and focus stimuli on the receptors.
   Examples: eye, cochlea, vestibular apparatus.
2. Complex sense organs: highly specialized receptor and capsule, located in relevant tissue in such a way as to determine response characteristics of the receptor.
   Examples: muscle spindle, taste buds.

A

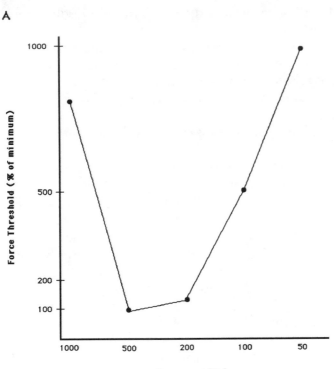

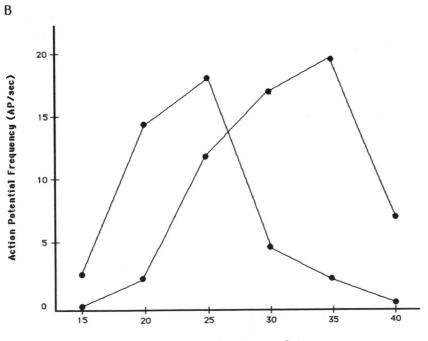

Figure 3-1. Sensory receptor tuning curves. **A.** Frequency tuning curve for a Pacinian corpuscle. **B.** Temperature tuning curves for two thermal receptors.

3. Complex encapsulated endings: specialized capsule that serves to determine response characteristics.
   Examples: Pacinian corpuscle, Meissner corpuscle, hair follicle receptor.
4. Simple encapsulated fibers: location and receptor membrane components serve to determine response characteristics.
   Examples: olfactory neurons, some thermoreceptors, Golgi tendon organs.
5. Free nerve endings: response characteristics determined primarily by location in tissue.

Receptors may respond either to stimuli only in their immediate locale or to stimuli that originate at some distance from the receptor. Teloreceptors respond to stimuli generated outside of the body. They include rods and cones of the retina, cochlear hair cells, and olfactory neurons. Exteroceptors respond to stimuli located on or immediately within the skin or the mucosa exposed to the external environment. They include many types of mechanoreceptors, thermoreceptors, nociceptors, and taste buds. Proprioceptors are so classified not only on the basis of stimulus location but also on the basis of having the stimulus generated by body movement or position relative to outside forces. They are located within the body and include muscle spindles, Golgi tendon organs, Pacinian corpuscles, joint mechanoreceptors, and vestibular hair cells. Enteroceptors also are located within the body and respond to stimuli arising in the body and relating to the viscera. They include mechanoreceptors, thermoreceptors, chemoreceptors, osmoreceptors, and nociceptors.

Proprioceptors are of particular importance to physical therapists because of their involvement in guiding skeletal motor activity. Muscle spindles and Golgi tendon organs will be discussed here in some detail; vestibular receptors will be described later (Chap. 9).

Muscle Sensory Receptor Anatomy

Skeletal striated muscle has two intrinsic sensory receptors: muscle spindles and Golgi tendon organs. Although other proprioceptors such as deep pressure receptors and joint motion sensors are important in the general reporting and regulation of muscle activity, the two intrinsic receptors appear to have primary importance in the autoregulation of skeletal muscle activity.

The muscle spindle is a complex, fusiform sense organ composed of specialized striated muscle (intrafusal fibers). It is one of the sensors having both afferent fibers and efferent or regulatory innervation, as summarized in Table 3-1. The intrafusal fibers can be one of two subtypes: nuclear bag fibers or nuclear chain fibers. The nuclear bag fibers are larger in diameter and have their nuclei clustered in the central region of the fiber; the thinner nuclear chain fibers have their nuclei more spread out in this region (Fig. 3-2).

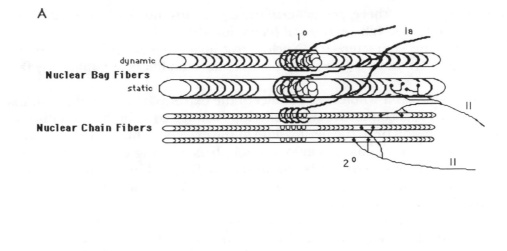

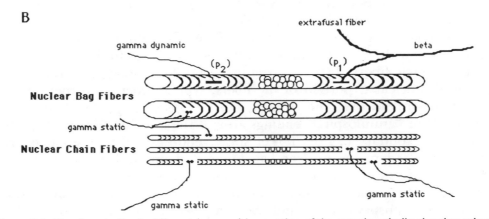

Figure 3-2. Muscle spindle. **A.** Afferent (sensory) innervation of the muscle spindle showing primary (1°) and secondary (2°) endings with their respective la and group II fibers; **B.** Efferent (motor) innervation of the muscle spindle showing plate$_1$ (p$_1$) endings for beta fibers, plate$_2$ (p$_2$) endings for dynamic gamma fibers and static gamma fibers ending on static nuclear bag fibers and nuclear chain fibers.

TABLE 3-1. Muscle Spindle Innervation

Intrafusal Fiber	Contraction Innervation Characteristics	Efferent	Afferent
Nuclear Bag			
dynamic	slow, dynamic	β, p$_1$ γ_d, p$_2$	la, 1° ending
static	fast, static	γ_s, trail	II, 2° ending
Nuclear Chain	fast, static	β, p$_1$ γ_s, trail	II, 2° ending

In most spindles, there are at least twice as many nuclear chain fibers as nuclear bag fibers. Like extrafusal fibers, intrafusal fibers have varying tension generating characteristics. Nuclear bag fibers may be either fast (static, b-2) or slow (dynamic, b-1) twitch type; nuclear chain fibers are uniformly fast twitch.

The spindle, as a whole, lies parallel to the extrafusal muscle fibers and is encapsulated in a connective tissue envelope connected at both ends either to the muscle tendon or to the perimysium of the extrafusal fibers. This arrangement permits length changes in extrafusal fibers to bring about corresponding length changes passively in the intrafusal fibers. These intrafusal fiber length changes may or may not be correlated with intrafusal fiber tension changes, as will be discussed later.

Spindles are located close to one or a few functionally related motor units. The relative density of spindles varies in different skeletal muscles. There appears to be at least some functional basis for the density of spindles: muscles with predominantly postural activity tend to have a higher density of spindles than muscles with predominantly ballistic activity.

The sensory, or afferent, innervation of muscle spindles consists of two types of fibers with characteristic anatomical relationships to the two types of intrafusal muscle fibers. Type Ia fibers have peripheral terminations around the central, nucleated portion of the fibers; type II fibers have peripheral terminations spread over the striated, polar regions. Type Ia fibers form primary (1°) or "annulospiral" endings around the intrafusal fibers. Type II fibers form secondary (2°) or "flower spray" endings. Primary endings are found on both dynamic nuclear bag fibers and on nuclear chain fibers. Secondary endings are located on static nuclear bag fibers and on nuclear chain fibers. There may be either a one-to-one or a several-to-one correspondence between sensory endings and fibers. A given afferent fiber may receive information either from just one type of intrafusal fiber or from both types.

The efferent innervation of muscle spindles also is varied and related to the type of intrafusal fiber innervated. In humans, the major innervation comes from two types of gamma motor neurons: static and dynamic. The static gamma fibers terminate in trail endings on static nuclear bag fibers and nuclear chain fibers. Dynamic gamma fibers terminate in plate$_2$ (p$_2$) endings on dynamic nuclear bag fibers. As with the afferent fibers, patterns of innervation may be quite varied: a given gamma fiber may innervate only one intrafusal fiber, several members of the same type of intrafusal fiber, or both nuclear bag and nuclear chain fibers. Additional motor innervation is supplied in some muscle through type beta efferents. Beta neurons, which are intermediate in size between alpha and gamma motor neurons, innervate both extrafusal and intrafusal fibers. The intrafusal innervation goes primarily to plate₁ (p₁) endings on nuclear bag fibers, although in some cases nuclear chain fibers may also be innervated. Beta innervation provides for "hard-wired" coactivation of extrafusal and intrafusal fibers.

Golgi tendon organs (GTOs) are simple encapsulated sense organs located among the connective tissue fascicles of tendons (Fig. 3-3). Their location in series with the contractile elements of skeletal muscle permits them to sense changes in muscle tension transmitted to the tendon. There appears to be some correlation between GTO placement in the tendon and entry of motor units into the tendon, permitting specific reporting of motor unit activity. Golgi tendon organs have only simple afferent innervation through type Ib sensory neurons.

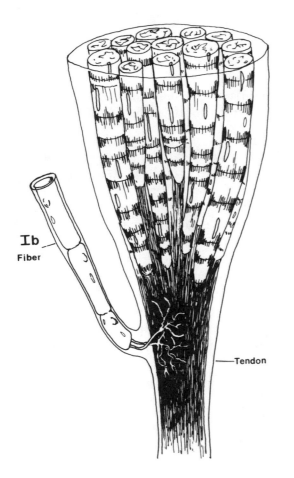

Ib
Fiber

Tendon

Figure 3-3. Placement of a Golgi tendon organ in a skeletal muscle tendon. The individual Golgi tendon organ is placed in such a way as to sense tension in a limited number of muscle fibers.

Review Exercises

3-1. Locate on the classification grid below the following receptors:

a. Pacinian corpuscle in dermis
b. retinal rod
c. olfactory neuron
d. osmoreceptor
e. thermal receptor in tongue
f. muscle spindle
g. hair follicle receptor
h. free nerve ending in wall of intestine
i. Golgi tendon organ
j. vestibular hair cell

	EXTEROCEPTOR	ENTEROCEPTOR	PROPRIOCEPTOR	TELORECEPTOR
CHEMORECEPTOR				
MECHANORECEPTOR				
THERMORECEPTOR				
ELECTROMAGNETIC RECEPTOR				
NOCICEPTOR				

3-2. Tuning Curves by personal experience. See if you can describe "tuning curves" or receptor sensitivity for the following:

a. chemoreceptors in taste buds on the front and back of your tongue
b. electromagnetic receptors in the lateral retina vs the fovea or central retina

3-3. Design a receptor. The modality and tuning curve of a receptor are determined by the ability of the receptor to be excited by certain stimuli, the structure of the capsule and the location of the receptor. Practice identifying the value of these factors by designing a new receptor.

a. Design a receptor which would be sensitive to nuclear radiation. Where would be the best place in the body to locate the receptor? What would it have to be responsive to? What type of capsule would it require, if any?
b. Birds have the ability to sense the orientation of magnetic fields. Humans lack this ability. Design a magnetic receptor which would permit humans to navigate in earth orbit using magnetic fields. Again, describe and justify the location of the receptor in the body, the mechanism it might use to sense magnetism, and the type of capsule which could be used.
c. There is considerable evidence that the human brain determines the location of fingers using information from receptors located in the skin rather than from joint or muscle/tendon proprioceptors. Design receptors which could serve this purpose. What stimuli would they need to be specifically responsive to? How would they be arranged in or near the skin?

4

Information Transfer

Conduction Within Neurons

Like all excitable tissue, neurons have the capabilities of excitation and conduction through the processes of charge and ion transfer. These processes may take the form of electrotonic conduction, regenerative conduction, or saltatory conduction, depending primarily on the morphological characteristics of the part of the neuron involved. Neurons, like all cells, have a difference in electrical potential between the inside and the outside of the cell at rest, with the inside being relatively negative. When the cell is activated, the potential difference may either decrease *(depolarization)* or increase *(hyperpolarization)*. In some types of activation to be discussed below, there is no measurable change in cell polarity, but there is a decrease in the facility with which the cell polarity may be changed, that is, the cell becomes relatively stabilized.

Electrotonic Conduction

In cable, or electrotonic, conduction, the transfer of charge along the neuron membrane is achieved through movement of ions along the membrane both inside and outside the cell (Fig. 4-1). Electrotonic conduction may involve either depolarization or hyperpolarization. Some movement of ions occurs through the membrane, with the result that over distance the change in charge at any point on the membrane decreases, leading to *degeneration* of the electrical signal. The rate of decrease in charge differential is described by the length constant (lambda) of the process, which is dependent on, among other things, the diameter of the process. The speed with which electrotonic conduction occurs is also dependent on the diameter of the process activated, being greater in larger diameter processes. Degenerative conduction is useful primarily in relatively short neuron processes, either dendritic branches or short axons. As a result of the ease with which charge differential at any point on the membrane can be varied, degenerative conduction is the optimal method of transferring charge when it is desirable to integrate or summate potential differences arriving at a point on the membrane from several differ-

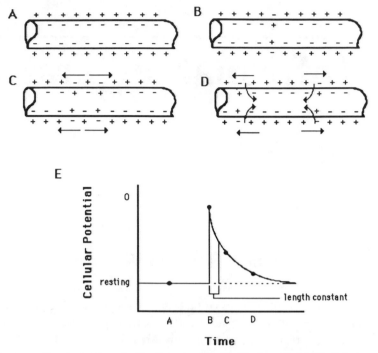

Figure 4-1. Electrotonic conduction. **A.** Resting charge distribution. **B.** Initial disturbance causing a change in charge distribution. Polarity may be locally reversed as indicated, or the cellular potential may simply move closer to O mv. **C.** Spread of depolarization in all directions from the point of initial disturbance. The area initially disturbed repolarizes. **D.** Level of depolarization decreases over time or distance due to ion movement through as well as along the membrane. **E.** Typical exponential decline in cellular depolarization over time (and distance) following initial depolarization. The length constant (λ) varies with the diameter of the fiber.

ent sources. Degenerative conduction, thus, is particularly useful in the dendrites and cell bodies of neurons receiving synaptic input from a number of sources. The changes in charge differential that are the basis for electrotonic conduction also are used in modifying neuron behavior near axon terminals as is seen in presynaptic inhibition and facilitation.

Regenerative Conduction

Action potentials are developed in long neuron processes. Typically, action potentials are developed in axons, but are found also in long dendrites, such as those carrying information from peripheral sensors to dorsal root ganglion cells. Action potentials have a constancy of amplitude that differs from that found in simple depolarization or hyperpolarization related to degenerative conduction (Fig. 4-2). Action potentials can be generated only when two conditions are met: The charge differential across the membrane is reduced to the point of threshold, and the membrane at that point has electrical characteristics that will permit the rapid flow of ions necessary to produce the reversal potential component of the action potential. Unlike electrotonic con-

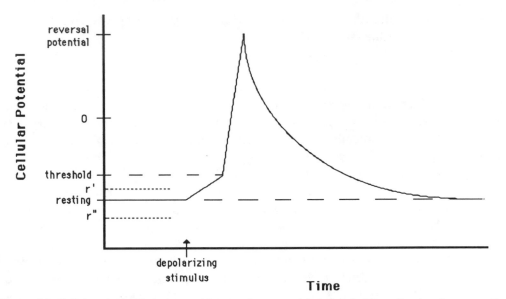

Figure 4-2. Cellular potential changes with an action potential. A depolarizing stimulus decreases the cellular potential to the threshold level at which point the regenerative (positive feedback) portion of the event is initiated. Note the change in slope of depolarization at threshold. Total action potential amplitude is the absolute value of the sum of the reversal potential value which is invariant for any given ion, and the resting cellular potential which may be normal (resting), partially depolarized (r') or hyperpolarized (r").

duction, action potentials always involve depolarization of the cell. Under most normal circumstances, the necessary bioelectrical characteristics to initiate an action potential are found only in certain places in the neuron, primarily in the axon hillock adjacent to the cell body; the terminal segment of sensory neuron dendrites; and at various places within the dendritic tree of neurons with large, complex dendritic trees. Once generated, however, the action potential will travel in all available directions along the neuron process; thus, action potentials generated at the axon hillock spread not only along the axon but back over the cell body and for a variable distance along the dendrites. The presence of an action potential in all parts of the neuron temporarily affects the changes in polarity resulting from synaptic action on the neuron. Axon potentials near the distal segment of sensory dendrites also spread in a retrograde direction depolarizing the distal segment itself. Depolarization of the neural membrane to the point of threshold can occur as a result of any of the following:

1. Decrease in charge differential that is due to the arrival of an electrotonic potential.
2. Change in ion concentration that is due to a change in the extracellular chemical composition.
3. Change in electrical characteristics of the membrane that is due to structural deformation.

4. Change in membrane components due that is to the presence of electro-magnetic radiation.

5. Change in charge concentration that is due to the presence of an electrical current.

Typically, only the first event is in a position to lead to the generation of action potentials. The next two events usually occur in relationship to the development of membrane depolarizations or hyperpolarizations that may then be conducted electrotonically. Retinal receptors sensitive to electromagnetic radiation do not normally generate action potentials. In humans, changing extracellular electrical fields certainly occur in the CNS, but their ability to bring about functional changes in neuron polarity has not been documented firmly. The introduction of electrical currents, of course, is used in clinical settings to cause artificial activation of neurons for evaluation or treatment purposes.

Action potential generation occurs at the axon hillock and the sensory terminal segment. At the axon hillock, there is integration or summation of electrotonically conducted depolarizations and hyperpolarizations of the membrane. With depolarization to threshold, an action potential is generated. The timing of arrival of the various changes in membrane polarity is of critical importance in determining whether an action potential will be generated.

The process of generating an action potential at a sensory terminal is termed *transduction* of the stimulus (Fig. 4-3). At a sensory terminal, electrotonically conducted changes in cell potential are summated either in the terminal portion of the process (in the case of unmyelinated fibers) or at the first node of Ranvier (in the case of myelinated fibers). Individual generator potentials from a single receptor may be summated temporally, or multiple generator potentials from several receptors innervated by a single neuron may be summated. The changes in cell potential in the terminal segment may

Figure 4-3. Flow diagram of the events involved in stimulus transduction.

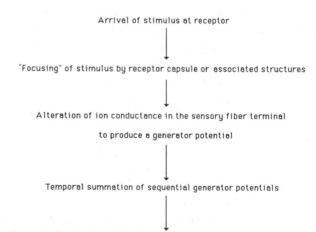

Arrival of stimulus at receptor

"Focusing" of stimulus by receptor capsule or associated structures

Alteration of ion conductance in the sensory fiber terminal to produce a generator potential

Temporal summation of sequential generator potentials

Depolarization to threshold of nerve process at point of lowest threshold

Generation of an action potential in the neuron

be caused by changes in extracellular ion composition or concentration, by structural deformation, by the presence of electromagnetic energy, or by changes in electrical behavior of the terminal segment as a result of changes in the thermal energy (temperature) of the immediate environment. Which particular change is normally responsible for the production of a generator potential in the terminal segment is a complex function of process location, capsule structure, and membrane characteristics. A generator potential caused by any of the effects listed above may either depolarize or hyperpolarize the terminal segment of the sensory neuron. Most sensors change polarity only in one direction, and only temporal summation of electrotonically conducted depolarizations is of importance in reaching the action potential threshold.

Saltatory Conduction

In situations where the distance to be covered by an action potential is great and the information being transferred must be integrated rapidly to support normal neurological function, the neural processes are myelinated. Myelin acts as an electrical insulator and limits the ability of the process to generate action potentials; thus, the potentials are generated only at the nodes along the process where the layers of myelin are thin or essentially nonexistent. The time required to move an action potential from one location to another along a membrane is only minimally dependent on the distance between active points under normal physiological circumstances, therefore an increase in the distance between active points serves to reduce the number of times the potential must be generated over a given length of process. The end result of myelination, therefore, is an increase in speed of transfer (conduction velocity) of the action potential from the point of its origin to its destination, or an increase in conduction velocity (Fig. 4-4). Conduction velocity, thus, is depen-

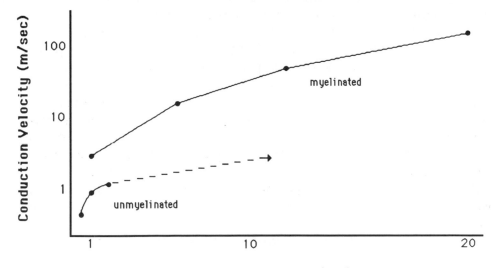

Figure 4-4. Conduction velocity dependence on fiber diameter and myelination.

dent on two factors: process diameter (which affects regenerative conduction as it affects electrotonic conduction) and the degree of myelination of the process. Myelinated processes include predominantly long, large-diameter processes; for example axons of the somatomotor system, dendrites of certain sensory receptors, and a variety of axons within the CNS. Myelination of long CNS dendrites has also been demonstrated.

Synaptic Transmission

The arrival of an action potential at a presynaptic terminal causes depolarization, which in turn causes a change in membrane permeability to calcium, leading to diffusion of calcium down its concentration gradient into the cell. The amplitude of the calcium flux is related directly to the change in membrane potential, which can be variable. Although an action potential for a given neuron is always of the same amplitude above threshold, the voltage difference between resting potential and threshold can vary depending on the presence of other hyperpolarizing or depolarizing changes existing in the presynaptic region. There is an additional direct relationship between the amount of calcium entering the presynaptic region and the amount of neurotransmitter released. Thus, alterations in resting potential in the presynaptic region can be a useful way of modulating synaptic activity. Figure 4-5 illustrates these synaptic events as they occur at the neuromuscular junction of the somatomotor system. Release of transmitter may be modulated further by repeated activation of the neuron; in some cells repeated activation can cause a potentiation of transmitter release (one component of what is termed "posttetanic potentiation"). If a neuron is activated regularly and rapidly over an extended period of time (much longer than that required for potentiation), the supply of neurotransmitter may be exhausted temporarily, and the synapse will demonstrate fatigue. Posttetanic potentiation is a normal physiological occurrence in the nervous system, with some information transmission processes depending on it. Synaptic fatigue, on the other hand, is pathological. Because calcium entry into the presynaptic region is dependent on depolarization of the membrane but not necessarily on the presence of an action potential, synaptic activity may occur in the absence of an action potential. In some neurons in which action potentials are not generated routinely, synaptic activity is dependent on the depolarization resulting from electrotonic depolarization of the neural processes. Synaptic activity among dendrites is an example of this type of synaptic activation. In most neurons, very small amounts of neurotransmitter are being released continuously in a random fashion, which probably is related at least in part to variations in intracellular calcium concentration.

Released neurotransmitters cross the synaptic cleft by the process of diffu-

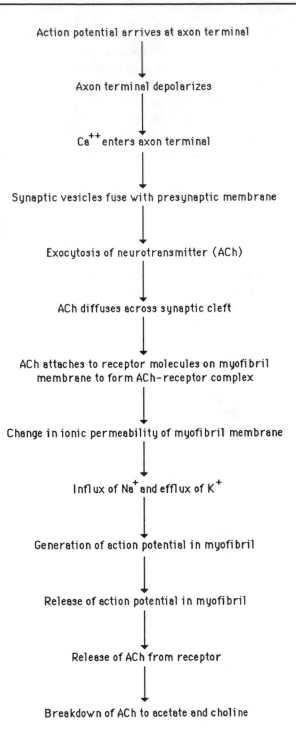

Figure 4-5. Flow diagram of synaptic transmission at the neuromuscular junction.

sion. Directionality is given to the movement by the relatively high concentration of neurotransmitter on the presynaptic side of the cleft and the relatively low concentration on the postsynaptic side resulting from transmitter uptake. Cleft morphology also assists in directing the movement of transmitter to the receptors on the postsynaptic membrane. Receptors for neurotransmitters may also be located on the presynaptic membrane, permitting uptake by the presynaptic cell, with subsequent modification of its activity. Combination of the neurotransmitter with the receptor molecule typically causes a change in protein configuration in the membrane leading to a change in permeability for one or more ions. The particular change in ion flux caused is dependent on both the neurotransmitter and the receptor; that is, a given transmitter may cause different changes in ion flux in postsynaptic cells depending on the nature of the receptor molecule. If the flux is such that there is a net increase in positive charge inside the cell, or a net decrease in negative charge, the cell will be depolarized at the synapse, or excited. If the reverse is true, the cell will be hyperpolarized, or inhibited (Fig. 4-6). The change in polarity is due to changes in flux of specific ions. The actual polarity change that will occur at any given time is dependent on the relationship between the resting cell potential and the equilibrium potential of the involved ion. If the two happen to be equal, no polarity change will be evident with the change in ion flux. Certain transmitters, usually classed as neuromodulators, can act on the membrane in such a way as to inhibit changes in ion flux. This action brings about stabilization of the membrane so that it is less responsive to subsequent inhibitory or excitatory transmission.

The time of action of neurotransmitters includes the latency time before the response begins and the duration of the response. These times vary from as short as 20 msec to as long as several minutes. Transmitters with long time courses are classed as neuromodulators. Various possible postsynaptic events and their time courses are outlined in Table 4-1.

Within the postsynaptic cell, the changes in membrane polarity caused by neurotransmitter action can summate, both temporally and spatially, and can be transmitted from one part of the cell to another by electrotonic conduction. Conduction of polarity change may occur in all directions from the point of synapse; in many cases, dendrite morphology enforces certain preferred routes on electrotonic conduction. As polarity changes are transmitted throughout the cell, some will die out before reaching all parts of the cell. Changes in synapse location, which can occur throughout life, take advantage of these characteristics of impulse conduction in dendrites. Such changes are theorized to be part of the microanatomical substrate for learning.

After initiation of the postsynaptic events, the neurotransmitter-receptor complex must be broken down or deactivated. Two basic classes of deactivation mechanisms exist:

1. Release of the neurotransmitter from the receptor with subsequent removal of the neurotransmitter either by enzymatic catalysis in the extracellular fluid or blood or by reuptake into the presynaptic cell followed by catalysis or functional recycling.

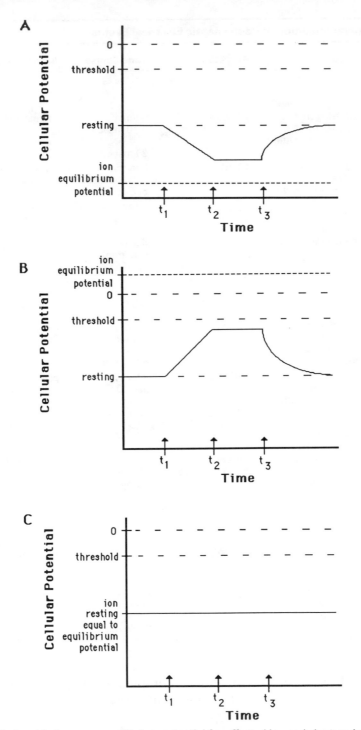

Figure 4-6. Relationship between equilibrium potential for affected ion and changes in cellular potential. **A.** The equilibrium potential for the affected ion is more negative than the current resting potential. Upon stimulation the cell is hyperpolarized. **B.** The equilibrium potential is more positive than the resting potential and the cell is depolarized. **C.** The equilibrium and resting potentials are equal and there is no noticeable change in cellular polarity upon stimulation although there is an increase in ion flux. In this situation additional potential changes are inhibited.

TABLE 4-1. Characterization of Postsynaptic Electrical Events

Event	Cause	Amplitude	Time Course	Ionic Changes
Excitatory Postsynaptic Potential (EPSP)				
fast-EPSP	AP-triggered release of neurotransmitter	20-50 mV	latency: 3-10 msec decay: 20 msec	increased Na^+, K^+ flux decay:
slow-EPSP	AP-triggered release of neurotransmitter	10 mV	latency: 100-400 msec decay: 20 sec	possible inactivation of K^+ flux
late slow-EPSP	AP-triggered release of neurotransmitter	10 mV	latency: 1-5 sec decay: 5-10 min	increased Na^+, K^+ flux
Inhibitory Postsynaptic Potential (IPSP)				
fast-IPSP	AP-triggered release of neurotrans-mitter	2-4 mV	latency: 3 msec decay: 5-25 msec	increased K^+ or Cl^- flux
slow-IPSP	AP-triggered release of neurotransmitter	2-8 mV	latency: 30-100 msec decay: 10-30 sec	possible change in some active ion transport
Pre-Synaptic Inhibition				
	AP-triggered release of neurotransmitter	variable, less than threshold	latency: 10 msec decay: 300 msec	increased Cl^- or Na^+ flux
Miniature Post-Synaptic Potential (miniature endplate potential, m.e.p.p.)				
	random release of quanta of neurotransmitter	0.5 mV	latency: 1-2 msec decay: 30-40 msec	increased Na^+, K^+ flux

2. Uptake of the receptor-transmitter complex by the postsynaptic cell with subsequent receptor recycling and transmitter catalysis.

Neurochemicals

The chemicals released at a synapse from a neuron may primarily have trophic effects on the recipient cell or primarily have information transmission effects. Undoubtably, some chemicals may have both types of effects.

Those having primarily information transmission effects can be further classified as being neurotransmitters, neuromodulators, or neurohormones. Differentiation among these classes is made on the basis of 1) the type and timing of the effect on the recipient cells and 2) the medium into which the chemical is released. The type of chemical itself is not a basis for classification because the same chemical can act in any of the three possible modes.

Neurotransmitters are chemicals that, when released by a presynaptic cell, have a specific and relatively brief effect on the electrical properties of a postsynaptic cell. For a chemical to be classed as a neurotransmitter, the following generally accepted criteria should be met:

Essential criteria:
1. The action of the suggested transmitter must be identical in every respect to naturally occurring synaptic activity.
2. The suggested transmitter must be released during synaptic activity in amounts adequate to account for the observed synaptic action.

Subsidiary criteria:
1. The suggested transmitter is present (stored) in presynaptic tissue in large amounts or
2. Enzymes necessary for synthesizing the suggested transmitter are present in the presynaptic cell, or both.
3. Specific mechanisms for deactivation of the suggested transmitter are present in the area of the synapse.
4. Action of the suggested transmitter can be blocked by specific antagonist agents (drugs) that effectively block naturally occurring synaptic activity.

Very few suggested transmitters meet these rather rigorous criteria. The action of acetylcholine at the neuromuscular junction, which has been studied most extensively because of its accessibility, is the only transmitter meeting all of them .

A neuromodulator is similar to a neurotransmitter, but it acts by facilitating or inhibiting the response of a postsynaptic cell to additionally present neurotransmitters; that is, it has a permissive action. The time course of neuromodulator activity (latency and decay) is considerably longer than the time course for neurotransmitters. Both of these observations suggest that neuromodulators act on postsynaptic cells primarily by second messenger systems within the cell, and they may have complex and extended effects on the electrical behavior of the cell. To be classed as a neuromodulator, a chemical must meet essentially the same criteria as exist for neurotransmitters, with the added complication that its interaction with known available neurotransmitters must also be taken into account.

Neurohormones differ from transmitters and modulators in that instead of being released at a synapse, they are released from an axon terminal directly into the circulation. From this point, they are transported through the circulatory system like any other hormone, interacting with appropriate target cells. The hormones of the posterior pituitary, or neurohypophysis, are all neurohormones, with their cells of origin located in the hypothalamus. Release of transmitter chemicals from axon terminals into the extracellular fluid or cerebrospinal fluid of the CNS has also been proposed as a means of generalized communication among certain sets of neurons. The appropriate classification of chemicals used in such a fashion is still debatable. Currently, they are referred to as neurotransmitters even though they are not released at a strictly defined synapse.

Neurotransmitters and the other two classes of information transfer agents are basically either protein or amino acid compounds or lipid derivatives. Pure carbohydrates have not been identified as transfer agents. Protein or amino acid transmitters can be classed as follows:

1. Peptides, either large or small:
   - large peptides including: substance P*, cholecystokinin, gastrin, and secretin;
   - small peptides including: neurohypophyseal releasing factors*, angiotensin, and endogenous opioids (enkephalins and endorphins)*.
2. Amino acids, including: L-glutamate*, L-aspartate*, glycine*, taurine, β-alanine, and ∂-amino butyric acid (GABA)*.
3. Amino acid derivatives, including:
   - catecholamines, primarily dopamine*, norepinephrine*, and epinephrine*;
   - others, primarily serotonin (5-hydroxytryptamine, 5-HT)* and histamine.

The major lipid derivatives functioning as transmitters include acetylcholine (ACh)* and prostaglandins. In the listing above, chemicals with asterisks are known to meet several, if not all, of the criteria for identification as neurotransmitters at particular synapses.

As mentioned above, the nature of the chemical is not an adequate basis for functional classification. In many instances, a given chemical may act in more than one capacity at different synapses, and in some cases it may act as both a transmitter and a modulator at the same synapse. The difference in function of transmitters at different synapses is dependent, of course, on the presence of different receptors. Examples of the varied effect of receptors on transmitter function are outlined in Table 4-2.

Synthesis pathways for neurotransmitters are determined during the process of differentiation of neurons and do not change for a given neuron after it has matured (Fig. 4-7). Any neuron may produce more than one neurotransmitter or modulator. Classically, it was thought that only one transmitter was released by a given neuron, and that this transmitter was released at all synapses formed by that neuron whenever the neuron was activated (Dale's law). More recent information strongly suggests that control of transmitter release is considerably more complex and subtle, with one neuron having the capability of producing and releasing a variety of transmitters or modulators at different synapses at different times. Nevertheless, many, if not all, neurons can still be characterized by the presence of one predominant neurotransmitter.

TABLE 4-2. Classification of Neurotransmitters by Postsynaptic Effect

Fast Postsynaptic Response	Slow Postsynaptic Response	Variable Response
Excitatory		
ACh	ACh	ATP
L-glutamate		dopamine
L-aspartate		5-HT
norepinephrine		histamine
substance P		
opiods		
Inhibitory		
GABA	GABA	taurine
glycine	norepinephrine	β-alanine
dopamine		ACh
ATP		
5-HT		
histamine		

A number of functional neuronal pathways have now been identified not only structurally and behaviorally but also by the presence of one or two specific neurotransmitters. This type of relationship between function and neurotransmitter used has long been known for the neuromuscular junction, which uses ACh, and the peripheral autonomic motor neurons, which at specific points use either ACh or norepinephrine. Examples of this type of relationship within the CNS include the descending pathways from the reticular formation of the brainstem which use serotonin, and some ascending

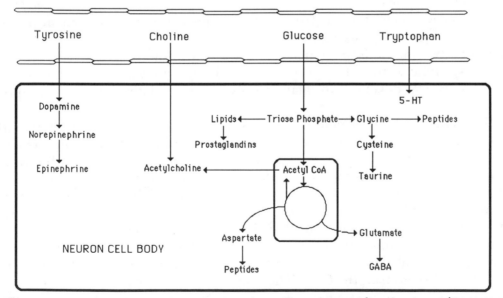

Figure 4-7. Synthesis pathways for neurotransmitters. The precursors for neurotransmitters move from CNS capillaries to the extracellular space without active transport. Processing of glucose through glycolysis and oxidative phosphorylation is essential for the production of amino acid transmitters.

pathways from the reticular formation, which use catecholamines. The best known CNS example is the dopamine system involving the basal ganglia. The growing body of information from neuropharmacological studies suggests that all functionally defined systems within the nervous system are probably identifiable by specific transmitter use. The economy of the nervous system also is illustrated by the use of the same transmitter in different systems. For this reason, one cannot use knowledge of the transmitter alone as a means for suggesting the function of a given neuronal system.

Basic Neural Networks

The basic unit of information transmission in the CNS, the synapse, can be organized into a number of simple networks used to handle a wide variety of types of information in various parts of the system. Several of these networks will be considered here. By combining these networks, very complex systems of information transmission can be created.

Secure networks or pathways are excitatory or inhibitory pathways in which the information is transmitted from one cell to subsequent cells in the network, with a high degree of certainty. Security may be ensured in a variety of ways:

1. Presence of synapses in places where the change in membrane polarity is most likely to affect the production of an action potential. Such locations include the axon hillock and immediately adjacent portions of the cell body and certain locations within dendritic trees.
2. Presence of multiple synapses between one presynaptic cell and the postsynaptic cell.
3. Convergence of axons from cells all transferring very similar information onto one postsynaptic cell.

The first two methods are generated frequently in the process of learning in which synaptic security for specific types of information is increased. Convergence may also develop with mature cells within a relatively limited synaptic zone.

The simplest type of neural circuit is one in which information is passed directly, without any modification, from one neuron to the next in a chain. Such a circuit allows for highly secure transmission of information but does not permit any modification of information. Interaction and information modification is permitted typically through the use of divergent and convergent circuits (Fig. 4-8). In *divergent* circuits, the synapses involved frequently have different degrees of security. Subsequent parallel circuits permit transmission of the same information but with differing types of modification. Divergent, parallel pathways can be used to synchronize neural activity in widespread regions of the CNS. The synchronized activity of cerebral cortical neurons during some stages of sleep is an example of normally occurring synchronization provided by these types of circuits. Very generally, sensory systems can be viewed as being predominantly divergent in character, spread-

A

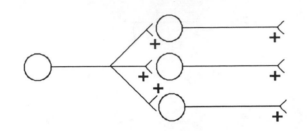

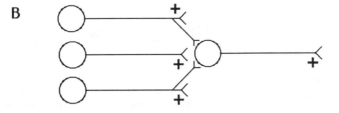

B

Figure 4-8. Divergent (A) and convergent (B) neural circuits.

ing a given piece of sensory information to a wide variety of processing centers within the CNS. Motor systems, on the other hand, can be viewed as essentially convergent, collecting information from a number of central sources for delivery to one or a few motor neurons.

Neurons may operate in either of two modes: inactive unless activated by synaptic input or spontaneously active. Alpha motor neurons are examples of cells that are inactive unless given synaptic (or stimulus) input. Spontaneously or cyclically active neurons do not have a stable resting potential but periodically depolarize to threshold in a manner similar to that seen in pacemaker cardiac muscle cells. Pacemaker type cells may be present in the brainstem in control centers for such cyclical activities as breathing. Entire neural circuits also may demonstrate cyclical activity (Fig. 4-9). This may be caused either by the presence of pacemaker cells within the circuit or by the cyclical input of outside information. Cyclical circuits may be of the re-entry type, involving at least two neurons, or of the recurrent type, in which an axon collateral synapses back on the original neuron. Recurrent circuits function primarily to regulate the activity in the involved neuron. Most central neural circuits maintain constant activity that may either be increased or decreased; very little evidence exists for circuits that are completely quiet until activated by outside information.

Inhibitory neurotransmission permits the use of inhibitory circuits (Fig. 4-10). Introduction of a single inhibitory neuron into a circuit simply decreases the probability of transmission of information through that pathway. When two inhibitory neurons are used in a constantly active series circuit, the second inhibitory neuron is inhibited by the first, in turn causing release from inhibi-

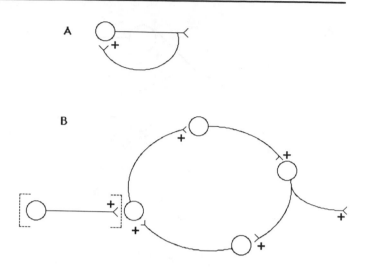

Figure 4-9. Cyclical neural circuits. **A.** Recurrent circuit in which the primary cell re-excites itself with a collateral axon. **B.** Re-entry type cyclical circuit. Repetitive activity may exist in such a circuit due to either the presence of a pacemaker cell within the circularly connected neurons or periodic excitatory input to the circuit from an external cell (in brackets).

tion of the following neuron. Parallel and divergent inhibitory circuits are used to permit enhancement of differences in information transmission. Combined divergent and parallel pathways permit the development of "surround" inhibition that serves to accentuate the differences in information between the parallel pathways. Cyclical inhibitory circuits can serve to regulate the timing of activity in the circuit.

Presynaptic modification of cell polarity is another effective method of controlling information transmission. Two basic types of presynaptic modification are known to exist: presynaptic inhibition and presynaptic disinhibition, or facilitation (Fig. 4-11). The timing of transmission and the latency and decay times of the postsynaptic potentials created are obviously of key importance in making these types of circuits work effectively. Both of these circuits were first studied in detail using primary afferents as the affected neuron. Presynaptic inhibition frequently is discussed or referred to as primary afferent depolarization (PAD). Presynaptic disinhibition is referred to as primary afferent hyperpolarization (PAH), although the affected neuron is not really hyperpolarized in the sense of being polarized beyond the level that would be seen in the totally unaffected fiber. Again, because of the use of primary afferents as the experimental material for study of this type of network, the changes in potential were recorded frequently from the dorsal roots. As recorded with extracellular electrodes, PAD causes a negative dorsal root potential, and PAH causes a positive dorsal root potential. It is now known that these types of networks occur in many other parts of the CNS.

Information Coding

Neural electrical impulses cannot contain information based on their amplitude. Electrotonic signals have an amplitude that varies with the diameter of the nerve fiber and the distance from the site of origin of the signal; action

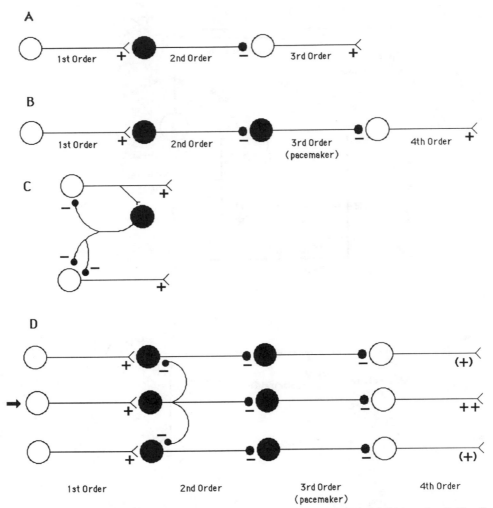

Figure 4-10. Inhibitory neural circuits. **A.** Simple inhibitory circuit. **B.** Double inhibitory circuit. The first order neuron excites the second order neuron which in turn inhibits the third order neuron. If the third order neuron is spontaneously active (pacemaker behavior) then activity in this entire circuit will result in effective dis-inhibition of the fourth order neuron. **C.** Re-entry inhibitory circuit with divergence (typical Renshaw cell circuit). **D.** Basic inhibitory surround circuit. Assume that the third order inhibitory neurons are pacemaker type cells. Activity in the central first order neuron will effectively dis-inhibit the central fourth order neuron. The divergent collaterals from the second order central inhibitory neuron create a triple inhibitory sequence on the lateral pathways, effectively increasing the inhibition on the fourth order neurons in these pathways. The end result is a significant difference in the level of excitation between the central and lateral fourth order neurons in the three pathways.

potentials have an invariant amplitude except when it has been affected near a nerve terminal by presynaptic modification. The meaning of information can be determined by two other characteristics of electrical signals: the identification of the synapse(s) being activated and the temporal pattern of occurrence of electrical signals. The first type of information coding generally is termed *location* coding, and the second is termed *frequency* coding.

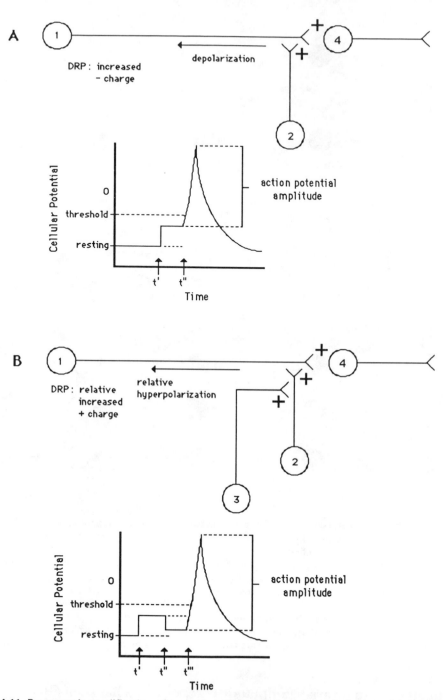

Figure 4-11. Presynaptic modification of synaptic activity. **(A)** Partial depolarization of the presynaptic region at t′ causes an effective decrease in action potential amplitude at t″ and thus in neurotransmitter release. **(B)** Inactivation of the presynaptic synapse by either presynaptic depolarization of neuron 2 (t″) or synaptic inhibition of neuron 2 can partially or wholly restore cellular polarity of neuron 1 to the resting level — relative hyperpolarization. The total amplitude of the action potential in neuron 1 at t‴ is thus increased. If neuron 1 is a spinal primary afferent a dorsal root potential which is negative for presynaptic inhibition and positive for presynaptic dis-inhibition can be recorded.

Location coding can be described on the basis of which neuron is active (labelled line coding) and which neuron is receiving the information (address coding). The concept of a labelled line or specific neuron (or nerve fiber) having information characteristics was first developed by Mueller in his doctrine of specific nerve energies. According to this theory, the modality and location of a sensory stimulus is determined within the nervous system by the identity of the active neuron. Experiments involving direct excitation of sensory neurons by electrical stimulation rather than by the use of naturally occurring stimuli have demonstrated that such labelled line coding does in fact serve to provide at least gross modality and specific location information in sensory systems. Motor systems also use location coding. This type of coding is of less value in specifying information in more complex integration systems within the CNS. Precise sensory submodality information and many other stimulus characteristics cannot be encoded completely by this method.

Address coding, in which there is a specific connection between sequential neurons, can code for modality and stimulus location in sensory systems and for specific muscle or muscle group activation in motor systems. It is also at least part of the basis for providing clues to information characteristics in complex integration systems. Many CNS pathways demonstrate "topographic" maps or their equivalent. A clear example of this type of coding are the sensory and motor homunculi that can be superimposed on the primary somatic sensory and motor regions of the cerebral hemispheres (Fig. 4- 12).

In frequency coding, information is contained in the frequency characteristics of action potentials (or electrotonic potentials). Frequency coding is useful in sensory systems for indicating modality and submodality, timing, and intensity of stimuli. In motor systems, frequency can specify intensity and

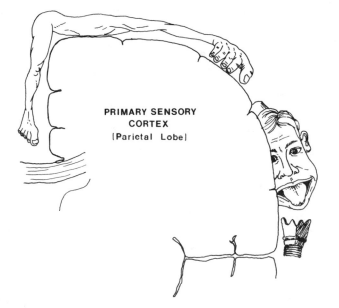

**PRIMARY SENSORY
CORTEX
(Parietal Lobe)**

Figure 4-12. Distribution of skin sensory projections to the primary sensory region of the parietal lobe (sensory homunculus). The size of body components indicates the relative area of cortex to which receptors from these components projects. Note the expanded size of the hand, face (particularly the mouth) and pharynx. A similar distribution (motor homunculus) can be displayed for the primary motor region of the frontal lobe.

other activation characteristics (eg, type of motor unit recruited) of effectors. Frequency coding typically does not carry spatial information such as sensory stimulus location or specific muscle activation. Responses of different mechanoreceptor primary afferents illustrates this type of coding (Fig. 4-13).

Sensory Receptor Field and Modification of Receptor-Afferent Behavior

Primarily because of capsule morphology and location of the receptor in the surrounding tissue, various receptors will have different types of receptive fields, (ie, the area and to a certain extent the characteristics of the stimulus) that will excite the receptor. Receptive fields may vary both in size and in uniformity. Additionally, many receptors are directionally specific, particularly receptors in the skin, the vestibular apparatus, and the retina (Fig. 4-14).

Receptor and primary afferent behavior may be modified in a number of ways, including the following:

1. Adaptation to a continued stimulus.
2. Availability of the receptor for stimulation.
3. Alteration of the sensitivity of the receptor.
4. Facilitation or inhibition of transmission of sensory information at synapses.

Receptors differ in their response to sustained stimulation. Nonadapting or slowly adapting receptors will generate multiple sequential action potentials in

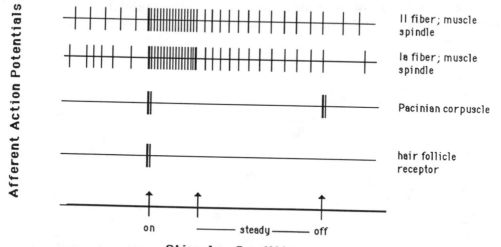

Figure 4-13. Basic mechanoreceptor coding patterns. Group II fibers show a regular resting discharge, a definite increase in frequency as stimulus intensity increases, and a steady, non-adapting discharge while the stimulus is steady. Group Ia fibers show an irregular resting discharge, an adapting response to a steady stimulus, and silence ("off" response) with stimulus release. Pacinian corpuscles are silent in the absence of a stimulus or during steady stimulus application and show a rapid burst of firing with stimulus application and release. Hair follicle receptors are similar to Pacinian corpuscles but show a response only to stimulus application.

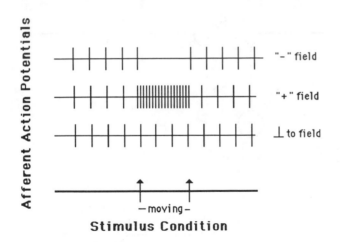

Figure 4-14. Directionally specific coding of receptors. Movement of a stimulus across the field in the one direction silences the afferent fiber ("−" field). Movement in the opposite direction causes an increase in afferent fiber firing frequency ("+" field). Movement directly perpendicular to the field causes no change in firing frequency.

response to a sustained stimulus. Adapting receptors produce one or only a few action potentials in response to onset or removal, or both, of a stimulus. Sensors that transduce information about stimuli that are typically momentary tend to adapt, even in the continued presence of the stimulus. Examples would be Pacinian corpuscles that respond to pressure, primary endings of muscle spindles, hair follicle receptors, and retinal receptors. The specific mechanisms underlying adaptation vary among receptors, but the end result in each case is a diminished or extinguished ability to produce generator potentials and thus action potentials.

The availability of a receptor for stimulation and alteration of receptor sensitivity require efferent control over the receptor or the surrounding tissue. Receptor availability is regulated frequently by reflex behavior; for example, changes in pupil diameter in response to variations in available light intensity, or withdrawal of an extremity from a painful stimulus. Generally speaking, teloreceptors and exteroceptors can have their availability controlled by more or less specific motor activity; interoceptors and proprioceptors lack this type of regulation. Relatively few receptors are subject to modification of their sensitivity. This type of control requires efferent motor control of some part of the receptor and typically is only available for receptors with complex capsules or those in complex sense organs. Examples include muscle spindles, retinal receptors, and cochlear hair cells.

Transmission of sensory information from the primary afferent to the remainder of the nervous system can be inhibited or facilitated in several ways, primarily gating and surround inhibition. Gating is the process of controlling the passage of information at a synapse. The regulation may occur either presynaptically through the mechanisms of PAD or PAH, or postsynaptically through integration of additional excitatory or inhibitory synaptic activity in the recipient neuron (Fig. 4-15). Gating is possible at every synapse in a sequential chain of information transmission. Surround inhibition uses various types of parallel inhibitory circuits. The main use of surround inhibition

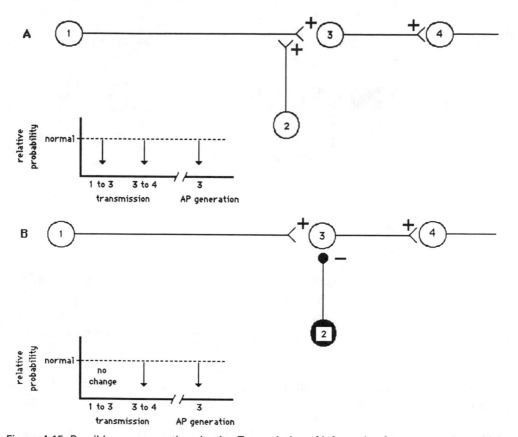

Figure 4-15. Possible synapse gating circuits. Transmission of information from neuron 1 to a higher order neuron can be gated or regulated either by presynaptic action of neuron 2 on neuron 1 **(A)** or by inhibitory synapses on higher order neurons **(B)**. In both cases the probability of transmission to neuron 4 is decreased. The effect of the synaptic activity on neuron 1 varies depending on the type of interaction.

is to increase the differences between information carried in parallel pathways. It can be used, among other things, for specifically delineating the receptive fields of sensory receptors.

Muscle Sense Organ Behavior

Muscle spindles and Golgi tendon organs can be used to illustrate several of the behaviors discussed for information transmission. Both of these sensors provide negative feedback regulation. Golgi tendon organs respond to changes in muscle tension in a very straightforward fashion, as might be expected from their relatively simple anatomy. The type Ib neurons are silent in the resting state and begin firing with the onset of tension in the tendon (Fig. 4-16). The firing rate increases with increased tension and remains constant with sustained tension. The GTOs appear to be more sensitive to active than to passive increases in tension, which may be explained by their close anatomical relationship to specific motor units.

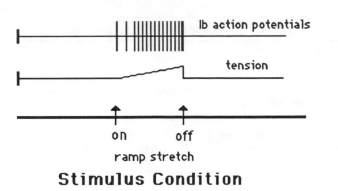

lb action potentials

tension

on   off

ramp stretch

Stimulus Condition

Figure 4-16. Golgi tendon organ response to increasing tension on a tendon.

Muscle spindles have complex response patterns to changes in muscle length. The basic response coding possibilities for a spindle (and for many other mechanoreceptors) are diagrammed in Figure 4-17. In general, a length-sensitive sensor, such as a spindle, may be responsive to changes in length itself or to changes in derivatives of length such as velocity and acceleration. Changes in length are referred to as static changes; changes in velocity or acceleration are termed dynamic changes. Valid sensing of static changes is a function of relatively stiff sensors, while more flexible sensors are better at recording dynamic changes. The central nuclear region of intrafusal

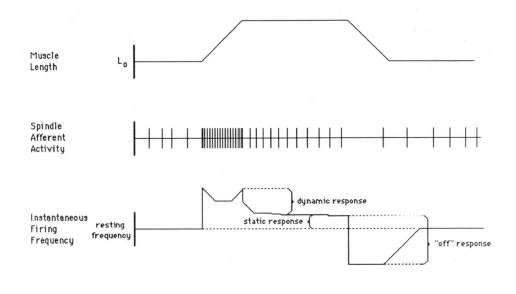

Muscle Length L_o

Spindle Afferent Activity

Instantaneous Firing Frequency   resting frequency

dynamic response

static response

"off" response

Time

Figure 4-17. Muscle spindle responses to passive changes in muscle length. The changes in instantaneous firing frequency are typical for each type of spindle afferent. Group Ia fibers from primary endings show definite initial, dynamic and "off" responses. Group II fibers from secondary endings show marked and constant (non-adapting) static responses and less noticeable initial, dynamic and "off" responses.

TABLE 4-3. Response Characteristics of Primary and Secondary Spindle Endings

Condition	Primary (Ia)	Secondary (II)
Resting Length	slow, irregular firing	moderate, regular firing
Initial Stretch	high frequency firing; frequency L_o dependent	moderate increase in frequency
Dynamic Response	high	low
Static Response	variable, possibly related to L_o	directly related to L_o
"Off" Response	definite; frequency drops to 0	moderate, length dependent; frequency may drop to 0

fibers, particularly nuclear bag fibers, is more flexible than the striated poles, thus leading to a greater sensitivity of primary endings and type Ia fibers to dynamic changes in muscle length. The secondary endings located over the striated regions are more sensitive to static changes. The stiffness of muscle spindles, and thus the sensitivity of the sensors, can be altered by actively contracting the intrafusal fibers in response to gamma (or beta) activation. Clearly, given the variety of afferent and efferent innervation patterns possible for spindles, an entire range of response patterns from purely static to purely dynamic is possible. The two extremes of response type are summarized in Table 4-3.

The presence of efferent innervation permits changes in response characteristics of the spindle sensors under different general conditions of muscle activation. An increase in static gamma activation generally causes an increase in the ability of the spindle as a whole to monitor static length changes. An increase in dynamic gamma activation increases the ability to monitor dynamic changes as illustrated in Table 4-4 and Figure 4-18.

Both Golgi tendon organ and muscle spindle sensory information are used to provide negative feedback control of skeletal muscle activity. The basic components of a neural system, as described in Chapter 1, can be linked to form feedback control systems (Fig. 4-19). Biologically, these systems are described as reflexes or responses to stimuli. All feedback systems have a resting or undisturbed level of outcome behavior activity and an activity level threshold at which a response to changes in behavior is initiated. In normal positive feedback systems, the response is to continue to change the level of outcome behavior activity in the same direction as the initial disturbance until

TABLE 4-4. Changes in Ia and II Spindle Afferent Responsiveness with Gamma Activation

Gamma Activity	Changes in Ia Fiber Response	Changes in II Fiber Response
Increased Gamma Static	decreased dynamic response increased static response decreased "off" response	overall increased firing frequency
Increased Gamma Dynamic	increased dynamic response increased overall firing frequency	minimal effect

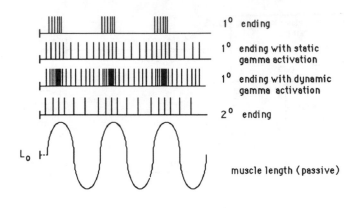

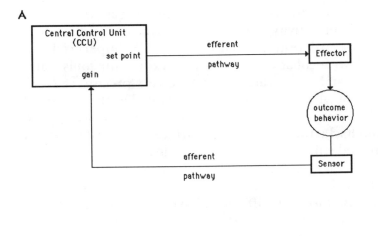

Figure 4-18. Primary and secondary ending (Ia and II) responses to passive sinusoidal muscle stretch and their changes with gamma activation. With static gamma activation Ia response becomes more "static" in character, while with dynamic activation the dynamic responses to stretch and the length sensitivity of the ending are both increased. Group II fiber response to static gamma activation (not shown) is a higher frequency of firing at all lengths.

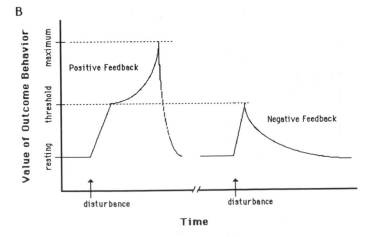

Figure 4-19. Basic negative and positive feedback control system responses. **A.** Elements of a feedback control system. System set point and gain are controlled centrally. **B.** Both negative and positive systems show a threshold for response to a disturbance in the value of the outcome behavior. When the value reaches threshold a positive system will respond to increase the change of value in the same direction as the initial disturbance until some maximum value is reached. At this point the system will permit the value to return to the resting level. In a negative system the response is to immediately start the return of the value to the resting level.

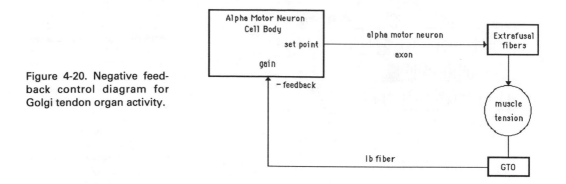

Figure 4-20. Negative feedback control diagram for Golgi tendon organ activity.

some maximum value is reached. At this point, recovery processes return the system to the resting level. In negative feedback systems, the response acts to start immediately returning the value of the outcome behavior to the resting level. Acting through the GTO negative feedback circuit, an increase in muscle tension through either active contraction or passive stretch brings about a negative feedback decrease in muscle contraction and a resulting decrease in tendon tension (Fig. 4-20). Similarly, an increase in muscle length, or specifically intrafusal fiber length, with passive muscle elongation results in an increase in extrafusal fiber activity and muscle contraction leading to a return of muscle length toward resting length (Fig. 4-21). Superficially, it would appear that these two feedback systems are working antagonistically. Their operation, however, can be integrated to provide very precise feedback control of muscle *stiffness* (Fig. 4-22). Stiffness can be defined as the degree of change of muscle length in response to a unit increase in externally applied muscle tension (delta t/delta l). Increased spindle afferent activity generally will bring about an increased stiffness; decreased spindle afferent activity will cause decreased stiffness. Golgi tendon organ activity itself is not subject to changes as a result of the lack of efferent regulation. The two basic types of spindle regulation can be used to alter stiffness behavior of muscle appropriately depending on the type of muscle contraction required (ie, relatively static as in postural activity or relatively dynamic as in ballistic activity) In addition, the sensitivity of the stiffness control system can be altered centrally, leading to changes in the threshold of the system. This is demonstrated peripherally by changes in the resting length (L_o) of the muscle (Fig. 4-23).

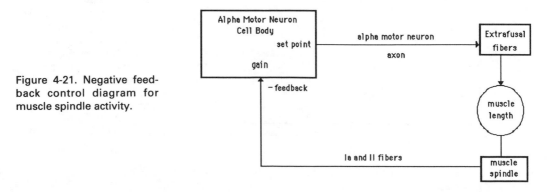

Figure 4-21. Negative feedback control diagram for muscle spindle activity.

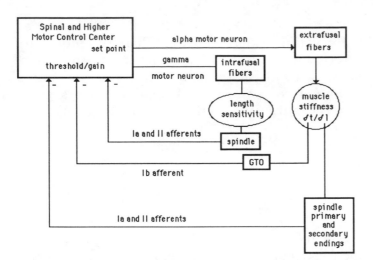

Figure 4-22. Negative feed-back control diagram for muscle stiffness. The enclosed gamma-spindle feedback loop is used to adjust the threshold and gain of the muscle stiffness system.

Figure 4-23. Changes in muscle stiffness regulation. The slope of the line expresses muscle stiffness. **A.** Changes in gamma efferent activity can effectively increase or decrease the gain of the system. With increased gain the muscle becomes more resistant to length changes and the slope of the line become steeper. With decreased gain the slope decreases. **B.** When there is a change in threshold of the entire regulatory system the slope of the line (stiffness) may be unchanged but the length setpoint (resting length of the muscle, L_0) shifts. Threshold changes may be brought about through changes in either gamma activation or level of alpha motor neuron excitability.

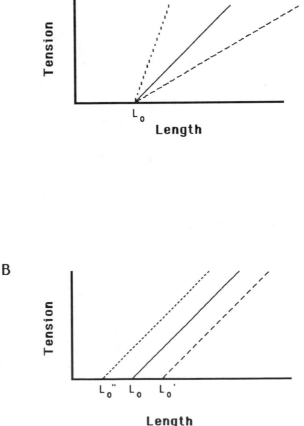

Review Exercises

4-1.   The receptive fields for various exteroceptive mechanoreceptors vary depending on the type of receptor and its location in the skin. Using a tool with two equally sharp (not dangerously sharp) points which can be adjusted to different separations (a common compass will work) determine the average size of skin pressure receptor receptive fields on the following locations:

- tip of the index finger
- tip of the nose
- dorsum of the forearm
- paraspinal skin

In all cases be sure to use a static rather than a moving stimulus.

The size of the receptive fields found on normal subjects represents the receptive fields for epicritic (discriminatory) touch. This information is carried by large diameter fibers in the periphery and by the dorsal columns in the spinal cord. Testing for receptive field size through two point discrimination is commonly used to determine the functional status of these fiber pathways.

4-2.   Amplify your design of receptors done in Chapter 3 to include specifications of the necessary receptive fields. In addition, indicate some basic network possibilities which could refine these receptive fields. Hint: inhibitory networks appear to be of considerable value in defining receptive fields.

4-3.   Use your current knowledge of possible neural circuits and of the components of the muscle spindle and Golgi tendon organ to design the most simple neural circuit which uses only labelled line and address coding and which will support the following observations:

- a. A muscle will contract in response to a rapid stretch stimulus.
- b. The antagonist of a rapidly stretched muscle will relax.
- c. A muscle will not contract in response to a slow stretch stimulus.
- d. A contracting muscle will relax when the tension on the muscle reaches a relatively high level.

Check your design with the information presented in Chapter 7.

4-4.   In myasthenia gravis the predominant symptom, skeletal muscle weakness, is caused by malfunction at the neuromuscular junction. On the basis of the following observations suggest what component of synaptic transmission is at fault.

- a. Distal latency (the delay time between motor nerve stimulation and EMG response) is normal.
- b. Muscle fatigue, as demonstrated both by a decrease in voluntary isometric tension production and EMG amplitude and frequency with electrical stimulation of the motor nerve, occurs much more rapidly than in a normal person.

c. Extracellular and intracellular calcium concentrations are within normal limits.
d. Acetylcholine is present in samples of synaptic extracellular fluid immediately following electrical stimulation of the motor nerve.
e. Administration of anticholinesterase drugs immediately relieves the weakness and fatigue symptoms.
f. There is evidence for a genetic basis for the disease.
g. There is evidence for an autoimmune component for the disease.

4-5.   Melzack and Wall proposed a theory of pain sensory transmission, now termed the gate theory, in which they suggested that transmission of pain information within the spinal cord is regulated by interaction between large diameter afferent fibers and the small diameter pain afferents. Diagram and discuss at least two networks which could produce such a gating effect.

4-6.   Sensory neurophysiologists have for many years used post stimulus time histograms—graphs, essentially, of the number of action potentials recorded from a single sensory afferent at sequential intervals following delivery of a stimulus—as a means of analyzing sensory coding of information. More recently, a similar type of analysis of action potential activity immediately prior to a motor act has been used in analysis of motor systems. What *assumptions* concerning neural coding of information underlie the design of experiments using this type of analytical tool?

4-7.   Functional models: Simple electronic circuits—or, for those with computer programming capability, computer programs—can be used to demonstrate some of the types of activity present in neural circuits. The following models can be made:
- convergent circuit
- divergent circuit
- parallel inhibitory circuit demonstrating inhibitory surround activity
- cyclical circuit with a pacemaker component

Presynaptic modification (PAH or PAD) can also be modelled. In such a model all the necessary electrical and chemical events need to be included.

5

Development, Degeneration, and Regeneration in the Nervous System

The nervous system as a whole is a derivative of the embryonic dorsal ectodermal plate that folds in to form the primitive neural groove. The neural groove closes dorsally to form the neural tube. Closure begins in the region that will form the brainstem and upper spinal cord at maturity and proceeds cranially and caudally. Developmental errors in closure lead to neural tube deficits (dysraphism) such as Arnold-Chiari syndrome (abnormal closure in the brain stem region) and various degrees of spina bifida (abnormal closure caudally).

The neural tube is divided early in development into three major concentric zones running the entire length of the tube: the ependymal, mantle, and marginal zones (Fig. 5-1). At maturity this basic division into zones is retained in modified form in the spinal cord, but it is not evident in the remainder of the CNS. Neurons develop from neuroblasts in the ependymal zone and migrate outward to their final locations in either the mantle zone or the marginal zone. Deep nuclei of the CNS develop in the mantle zone; cortical layers develop in the marginal zone. The movement of neurons is guided by flexible templates formed from glial cell processes. The timed chemotaxic interaction between neurons and glia is an essential component in neural development. Migratory patterns of cells into these zones is not always straightforward; for example, the pattern of migration in the cerebellar cortex involves movement of neurons both outward and inward through the marginal zone, following the movement of the template glial cells. Once

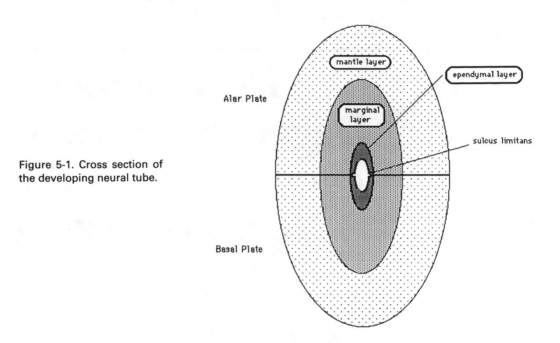

Figure 5-1. Cross section of the developing neural tube.

migration into the appropriate zone has been completed, functional differentiation of the neurons and synaptogenesis proceeds.

The neural tube is divided additionally throughout its length into a dorsal *alar* plate with predominantly sensory function and a ventral *basal* plate with motor function (Fig. 5-1). This basic division is clearly evident at maturity only in the grey matter of the spinal cord, but it can be traced to a certain extent in the brainstem as well. The dividing line between these two sets of cells is the sulcus limitans. In the cranial portion of the neural tube, the alar plate overgrows the basal plate and gives rise to the diencephalon and the cerebral cortex. A dorsal and ventral division in these complex areas, however, still exists. The motor portions of the diencephalon (primarily the hypothalamus) and the deep motor nuclei of the cerebral cortex both arise from ventral portions of the alar plate in this region. In the region of the brain stem, migrating groups of cells from the alar plate give rise to both the cerebellar cortex and the deep cerebellar nuclei. From this it can be seen that alar plate neurons give rise to cells that may have extensive integration and higher-level motor function as well as sensory function.

During development, the very extensive division and growth of cells in the anterior portions of the neural tube cause structures derived from these portions to overgrow the original tube greatly, and to become folded upon each other (Fig. 5-2). The neural tube can be divided into four primary anterior-posterior subdivisions: 1) the prosencephalon, 2) the mesencephalon, 3) the rhombencephalon, and 4) the spinal cord. The prosencephalon develops to the greatest extent, giving rise to the telencephalon, which includes the cerebral hemispheres and their deep nuclei and the rhinencephalon (olfactory

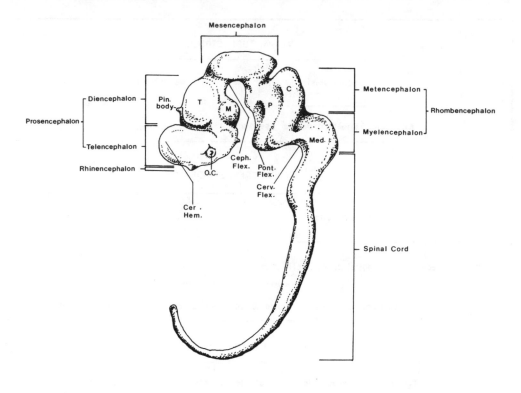

7 WEEKS

Figure 5-2. Central nervous system of a 7 week fetus. *C,* cerebellum; *Cer. Hem.,* cerebral hemisphere; *M,* mammillary bodies; *Med.,* medulla; *O.C.,* optic cup; *P,* pons; *Pin. body,* pineal body; *T,* thalamus.

and limbic cortex), and to the diencephalon, which includes the thalamus, epithalamus, hypothalamus, and posterior pituitary. The mesencephalon gives rise only to the midbrain of the brainstem. Between the prosencephalon and mesencephalon, there is a major bend in the primitive neural tube: the cephalic flexure. The rhombencephalon gives rise to the metencephalon and the myelencephalon. At maturity, the metencephalon includes the cerebellum and the pons of the brain stem; the myelencephalon becomes the medulla. A second major bend, the cervical flexure, occurs at the junction of the myelencephalon and the spinal cord. The spinal cord retains a primitive segmented pattern at maturity, showing specialized, enlarged development only in the segments related to the nerve plexi innervating the extremities.

Derivation and Maturation of Cell Types

All cell types in the central and peripheral nervous system (except cells of the dura and peripheral nerve covering tissues) are derived from three primary sources, two of which are ectodermal and one of which is mesodermal (Fig. 5-3). The first ectodermal source is neural tube ectoderm, which forms the original neural tube. The second ectodermal source is the neural crest,

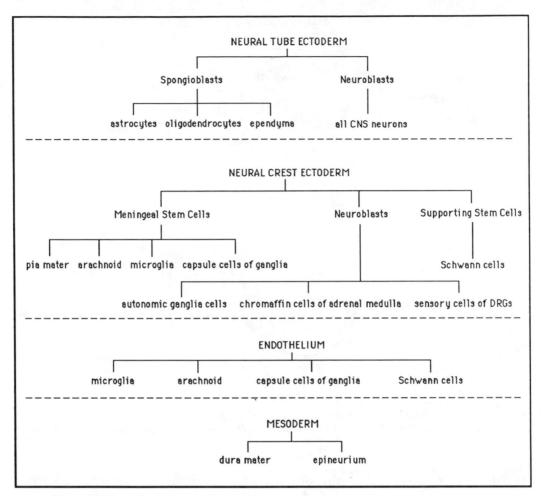

Figure 5-3. Cell lineages for the nervous system.

which forms dorsolaterally on both sides of the closing neural tube. The mesoderm supplies cells by way of the circulatory endothelium. All neurons are derived from ectoderm by way of either the neural tube that gives rise to all the neurons with cell bodies in the CNS or the neural crest that gives rise to all the neurons with cell bodies in the PNS. The supporting cells of the CNS and PNS are derived from all three basic sources; some may be derived by more than one route. Cells of the arachnoid and pia mater are derived from the neural crest.

Neurons and supporting cells develop to maturity through a number of processes; neurons retain the potential for only a few of these at maturity. The processes maintained at maturity are responsible for the ability of the nervous system to learn new behaviors and the ability of neurons to regenerate following injury. The developmental processes available to the immature neuron are listed below (those in italics are retained at maturity):

1. Division.

2. Differentiation.
3. *Growth.*
4. Migration (retained at maturity only for astroglia and microglia).
5. *Development of functional contact with other cells (eg. synaptogenesis and myelination).*

These developmental processes are subject to regulation by a number of factors, all of which are interdependent. Intrinsic to each cell is the genetic material. Differential expression of genetic information is brought about by the presence of chemicals in the local extracellular environment, the presence of microanatomical structure provided by adjacent cells, and the presence of trophic factors and synaptic activity at developing synapses. Timing is extremely important in differential genetic expression in neurons. Some genes can only be activated sequentially, and the induction effect of external messengers can occur only at certain specific times during development. The great importance of timing is demonstrated by the loss of the ability to differentiate at maturity. Chemical regulatory factors in the local environment, such as cell surface adhesion molecules, trophic chemicals released from neural (and possibly glial) processes, and neurotransmitters released at synapses, may have very specific, precise effects on a given developing cell. Intracellular fluid ion concentrations and pH can have a more general effect on a whole population of cells in a given region.

The importance of microanatomy in regulating development can be illustrated by the role of glia in the developing cerebellar cortex (Fig. 5-4). Migrating glial cells provide a continually changing template that guides the extension of processes of the cortical neurons and the migration of cell bodies. When the glial template is disrupted or lacking, normal cortical cell layer patterns do not develop, nor do normal synaptic patterns among the neurons.

Gross Changes in the Central Nervous System

Fetal Development

All of the potential developmental processes are occurring during fetal development. Rapid cell division, particularly during the first 22 weeks of gestation, causes a great enlargement of the telencephalon and rhombencephalon, particularly the cerebral and cerebellar hemispheres. By the age of 22 weeks, enlargement of the cerebral hemispheres has extended to the point where two major infoldings (fissures, sulci) are evident: 1) the Sylvian fissure lying nearly in the horizontal plane and separating the temporal lobe from the superior frontal and parietal lobes and 2) the central sulcus in the coronal plane separating the frontal and parietal lobes. On the midsagittal surface, the cingulate sulcus in the frontal and parietal lobes and the calcarine fissure in the occipital lobe also are evident. The CNS in a viable preterm infant (28 weeks) shows the development of additional sulci, but the overall aspect of the surface of the hemispheres is still very smooth compared with that of the full-

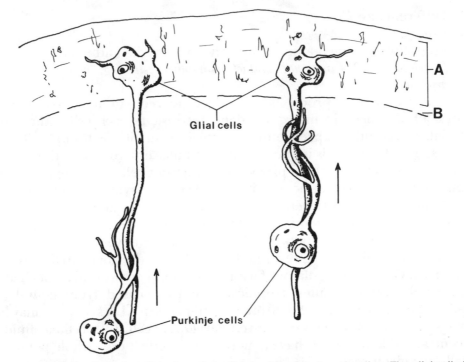

Figure 5-4. Cerebellar Purkinje cells using glial cells as a template for migration. The glial cells have already migrated to the molecular layer *(A)* of the cerebellum, leaving projections behind. The Purkinje cell on the left has made initial contact through a growth cone at the tip of one process. The Purkinje cell on the right is migrating along the glial process toward the final termination point in the Purkinje cell layer *(B)*.

term infant. At full term, the cerebral hemispheres have all of the sulci that will be present during maturity. The cerebellum is developed less completely: all sulci are present, but the overall volume is relatively small.

In addition to the growth in CNS volume and cell number during fetal development, neuron migration is occurring. By 36 weeks (full term) migration is essentially complete in all areas of the CNS with the exception of the cerebellar hemispheres. In this region, migration is not complete until the age of approximately 2 years. Development of functional contact, both synaptogenesis and myelination, follows the completion of migration. Synaptogenesis of most circuits is functionally complete at full term, except in the cerebellum, but it can and does continue, first at a rapid and then at a slower rate during childhood and maturity. Myelination is only minimally present at full term and continues through the first few years of infancy and childhood. The lack of myelination is most noticeable in the large diameter fiber tracts, explaining the relatively small size of such structures as the pyramids of the brain stem at full term.

Development During Childhood and Maturity

At birth the processes of cell differentiation, cell division, and cell migration, except in a few instances, are no longer present. Further development of the CNS is due to development of synaptic contacts, growth of existing cell processes, and myelination. All of these events continue to occur rapidly within the CNS during the first four to five years of childhood, by which time myelination and major cell process growth are essentially complete. Growth of processes continues in the form of elongation to match the overall growth of the body, particularly in the spinal cord and the PNS.

Development and change of synapses occurs throughout life. Synaptogenesis is correlated strongly with changes in the patterns of transfer of information within the nervous system; therefore, synaptogenises is correlated with all known types of permanent learning. The processes involved in synaptogenesis and microgrowth of neural processes are the basis for neural functional plasticity. The plasticity of the nervous system is greatest during fetal and early childhood development, but it continues throughout life. Microgrowth of processes related to synaptogenesis continues as long as synapse modelling is taking place.

Development During Senescence

The senescent brain shows gross changes related to loss of volume, primarily a widening of sulci. The loss of volume is due to both a loss of neurons (and glia) and, to a lesser extent, a decrease in myelination in some fiber pathways. The loss of neurons is related to the ongoing neuron cell death that begins during the fetal period and continues throughout life. This nonpathological cell loss appears to be related to changes in synaptic (and probably trophic) relationships among neurons as a result of the refinement of neural pathways, with a concomitant reduction in redundancy of synaptic connections. Insufficient studies of senescent brain plasticity have been done to document with certainty the degree of synaptogenesis and microgrowth function retained at this stage, but it is clear that in the nonpathological brain such functions are still present.

Disorders of Development

The many developmental disorders that may affect the nervous system can be related to the basic functions normally occurring during fetal development, specifically the following:

1. Disorders of cell division: production of less than normal numbers of neurons either overall or in discrete regions of the CNS, producing, for example, lissencephaly (a lack of development of sulci and gyri), arhinencephaly (lack of development of the rhinencephalon), and microcephaly.
2. Disorders of neural tube closure and ventricular system development, producing, for example, spina bifida, holoprosencephaly (lack of division of the cerebrum into two hemispheres), and hydrocephalus (lack of development of normal cerebrospinal fluid circulatory passageways).
3. Disorders of migration, giving rise to development of cell types in regions inconsistent with normal synaptogenesis.

In some developmental disorders, more than one basic function may be affected. As can be imagined, any disruption of cell differentiation, growth, or migration will give rise to abnormal synaptogenesis. Due to the different time of development of the various functional systems within the CNS, many development problems are both system and time specific.

Neural Degeneration and Regeneration

The processes that occur in neurons following a lesion of any part of the cell are dependent on the nature and extent of the lesion, the location of the lesion in the cell, and the extent to which the lesion affects the ability of the cell body to remain in functional connection with the cell processes. An understanding of neural protein synthesis and transport processes is helpful in understanding neuron reaction to injury.

Neural Protein Synthesis

Proteins synthesized by neurons fall into three main classes generally found in all cells: cytosol proteins, intrinsic membrane proteins, and secretory proteins. In neurons, however, the relative proportion of secretory proteins is higher than is found in other noncommunicating (nonsecreting) cells, and a great diversity of neural proteins exists both within and among neurons. Protein synthesis in neurons follows the same basic steps found in other cells:

1. Transcription of genetic material in the nucleus (or mitochondria).
2. Protein synthesis on either polysomes (for cytoplasmic proteins) or rough endoplasmic reticulum (Nissl material).
3. Enzymatic modification such as hydrolysis or addition of various chemicals (eg, glycossylation) in the smooth endoplasmic reticulum and Golgi apparatus.
4. Packaging in the Golgi apparatus for delivery to membranes or for exocytosis.
5. Translocation to the final functional site.

The main difference in this process between neurons and other cells is the extended translocation distance required for movement of protein and other cellular constituents from the cell body to the functional regions of dendrites or axons.

Neural Transport

Transport of proteins and other materials within the neuron takes place through two primary mechanisms termed *slow* and *fast* transport. Both of these mechanisms can be directed away from the cell body (orthograde or anterograde transport) or toward the cell body (retrograde transport). Microtubules in neural processes appear to be associated with fast transport, which occurs at a rate of 200 to 400 mm/day (orthograde faster than retrograde). Materials transported by fast mechanisms include the following:

1. Orthograde: peptide neurotransmitters, membranous organelles including synaptic vesicles, and trophic factors.
2. Retrograde: lysosomes and other organelles or materials to be broken down, and trophic factors entering the cell.

Additionally, nonphysiological entities entering the neuron can be transported toward the cell body by fast mechanisms. These include pathogens, such as herpes simplex and probably polio myelitis virus, and exogenous materials, such as horseradish peroxidase, which is used widely for tracing nerve pathways.

Slow transport is associated with microfilaments and can be subdivided into two classes with differing rates of movement. The slower class (rate 0.5-3 mm/day) transports primarily proteins related to the cytoskeletal elements of the neuron. The intermediate class (rate up to 6 mm/day) transports a variety of entities including mitochondria, cytosolic enzymes, and a few cytoskeletal elements including actin.

The events occurring following injury to a neuron cause loss of normal synaptic and trophic function at sites distal to the lesion and either regenerative activity or death in proximal sites including the cell body. A lesion is any disruption of microstructure sufficient to alter cellular function or any pathological change in cell function. (Fortunately for experimental science, penetration of a neuron cell body or a large neuron process by microelectrodes does not typically constitute a lesion if done with proper microtechnique). The events following a lesion can be summarized in the following steps, which may occur sequentially or simultaneously:

1. Loss of synaptic function distal to the lesion site.
2. Loss of transport past the lesion site.
3. Reorganization of structure and function within the cell body, with the end result of increased synthesis of proteins for cellular repair.
4. Degeneration and phagocytosis of the process distal to the lesion site.
5. Degeneration and phagocytosis of the proximal process near the lesion site and for a variable distance proximally.
6. Regeneration of the process and re-establishment of synaptic function.
OR
7. Neuron death or permanent degeneration to a dysfunctional state.
8. Transneuronal degeneration in postsynaptic cells (orthograde transneuronal degeneration) or presynaptic cells (retrograde transneuronal degeneration).

Neuron death is the probable outcome if the lesion is close to or in the cell body. Process regeneration will occur following relatively distal lesions, if all the required substrate for regeneration is available. Transneuronal degeneration is the result of loss of release of trophic factors as well as neurotransmitters from the initially damaged neuron. The bidirectional nature of this event reinforces the concept of release of trophic substances both in the direction of predominant synaptic transmission and contrary to it.

Degeneration of Process Terminals

When a process is severed from the cell body, the process terminals will degenerate. If the process is efferent (typically an axon), degeneration will involve loss of release of neurotransmitters and loss of trophic function. Loss of synaptic function is immediate following an axon lesion. The time of loss of trophic function has not been documented as clearly but is also likely to occur immediately. The terminal becomes separated from the remainder of the degenerating process, and the organelles in the terminal are disrupted. Surrounding supporting cells (glia or Schwann cells) phagocytize the remaining material.

Transneuronal Degeneration

Following loss of either an efferent (axon) or afferent (dendrite) process, the cells with which the degenerating cell made contact may also degenerate. This transneuronal degeneration is due to loss of both trophic and neurotransmitter input. In the CNS transneuronal degeneration involves the loss of associated neurons. The extent of transneuronal degeneration occurring following a given neuron lesion is dependent on the number of synapses involved in the lesion and the functional security of the affected synapses. An increasing level of synapse security tends to correlate with an increasing probability of transneuronal degeneration.

In the PNS lesions of axons of alpha and gamma motor fibers typically lead to degeneration of the innervated extrafusal or intrafusal fibers of skeletal muscle, unless reinnervation intervenes. Smooth and cardiac muscle typically does not degenerate following loss of autonomic motor innervation. These types of muscle are capable of independent excitation and are apparently less dependent on neurotrophic factors for their maintenance. Lesions of afferent fibers in the periphery also lead to "transneuronal" degeneration of the associated sensory receptors. The special cells forming end organs tend to degenerate in the absence of innervation, but they can either be regenerated following reinnervation or, in some cases, have new end organs formed from relatively undifferentiated cells in the area. The degree of reestablishment of sensory function appears to be closely related to the degree of specialization of the end organ: free nerve endings usually regenerate with no difficulty, but muscle spindles rarely regenerate effectively.

The PNS has an advantage over the CNS in reinnervation and regeneration of transsynaptic cells in that the peripheral innervation is not as synaptically specific. For example, in skeletal muscle, adequate reinnervation can occur through regrowth of the damaged axon, sprouting of adjacent undamaged axons, or a combination of the two processes. In the CNS, reinnervation by adjacent axons may serve to maintain cell viability, but the information transfer function of the cell is almost always altered significantly or lost.

Wallerian Degeneration

The events occurring within the lesioned process itself are termed Wallerian degeneration. The entire portion of the process distal to a lesion degenerates, but only a relatively short length of the process proximal to the lesion is affected. Wallerian degeneration involves segmenting of the process into small units, with internal disruption of all organelles present. Clearly, neuron transport ceases immediately with the onset of structural lesions. The degenerating process segments undergo phagocytosis by adjacent supporting cells: Schwann cells in the periphery and various available glia in the CNS. Myelin-producing cells, either Schwann cells or oligodendrocytes, reorganize their cell membranes to initially remove the myelin sheath and later prepare for manufacture of a new sheath. In the PNS, the cell bodies of the Schwann cells tend to remain in place and, in conjunction with the endoneurial cells, provide a template for regrowth of the neural process from a growth cone. In the CNS, the glia typically overgrow the ends of the neural growth cones, forming a glial scar. This glial scar formation, coupled with slight retraction of the lesioned nerve process, is one of the main obstacles to nerve regeneration following CNS trauma. The supporting cells, at least in the periphery, also release trophic factors that facilitate the formation and extension of the neural growth cone. There is an apparent absence of such trophic factors in the CNS glial cells at maturity. Current experimental approaches to the problems of limited regeneration in the CNS include the transplantation of embryonic cells of appropriate type that still have the capability of extensive process growth and synapse formation and the implantation of portions of peripheral nerve. Transferred peripheral nerve loses its own processes through degeneration, but the endoneurial tube and the remaining Schwann cells provide a pathway and biochemical support for the regeneration of central neural processes.

Growth of neural processes occurs at an average rate of 1 mm/day in the PNS. Remyelination of successfully regenerated nerve processes is a relatively slow process that does not begin until nerve process regeneration is nearing completion. Overall, although nerve process degeneration occurs rapidly and is typically complete within a few days to a week following injury, the regeneration process takes much longer, lasting several months to a year depending on the length of the process to be regenerated and the degree of myelination normally present.

Changes in the Cell Body of Lesioned Neurons

The changes in the cell body of a lesioned neuron, which have collectively been termed *Nissl degeneration*, or chromatolysis, are in fact not so much degeneration events as changes in function related to the need to manufacture the large amounts of structural material required for regeneration of processes. The types of proteins required are different, at least in proportion, to those needed during normal function. As a result, a change occurs in genetic activation and in endoplasmic reticulum function. Associated with these functional changes are changes in the morphology and the histological staining properties of the nucleus and the endoplasmic reticulum. The nucleus assumes an eccentric position, moving closer to the site of origin of the dendrites. The endoplasmic reticulum loses the ability to bind the chemicals typically used in Nissl type staining of neurons, hence the term "Nissl degeneration" because these staining techniques no longer demonstrate the presence of the reticulum. As regeneration of the processes occurs, the cell body resumes a more normal appearance.

Demyelination

The loss of the myelin coating of processes in either the CNS or PNS leads to a variety of functional abnormalities including the following:

1. Increased sensitivity of the process to electrical activity in adjacent fibers (cross talk).
2. Slowed conduction velocity.
3. A loss of trophic or metabolic support from the Schwann cell or the oligodendrocyte.

The changes in conduction velocity and sensitivity bring about alterations in function of the affected neuron; the loss of trophic support from the Schwann cell or the oligodendrocyte can lead to process degeneration and the formation of glial scars (as occurs, for example, in multiple sclerosis).

Neuromuscular Junction Degeneration

In the special case of the neuromuscular junction, loss of muscle activity follows the steps outlined in Figure 5-5. With loss of neurotransmitter and neurotrophic input from the alpha motor neuron axon, the muscle cell experiences "up-regulation" of the neurotransmitter receptors, with a loss of location specificity. As a result, the entire cell surface becomes more sensitive to the presence of acetylcholine. This change in sensitivity, coupled with other changes in membrane electrical behavior, are the probable basis for the presence of spontaneous electrical and contractile activity, or fibrillation, in individual denervated muscle cells. At the same time, there is a loss of the motor point for the muscle. In response to the loss of trophic factors, the muscle cell in turn releases chemicals that activate the branching of adjacent intact axons to provide reinnervation. These chemicals also assist in directing the regrowth of nearby growth cones of lesioned axons. Reinnervation by adjacent axons can lead to the development of larger than normal motor units in the muscle, which can be demonstrated as giant potentials in an electromyographic examination.

In the absence of reinnervation from either adjacent or regenerating axons, the muscle cell eventually will lose its contractile proteins and be replaced by a connective tissue scar (denervation atrophy). Fibrosis of denervated muscle can be delayed for extended periods of time (several months), although not indefinitely, by artificial activation through electrical stimulation. This type of intervention is of value in maintaining the viability of muscle tissue under circumstances of expected delayed reinnervation.

Skeletal muscle also will atrophy in the presence of intact but unused alpha motor neuron innervation. This disuse atrophy involves loss of contractile proteins, but it typically does not terminate in the development of fibrosis unless it is extended over a period of years. The presence of trophic factors from the intact axon apparently is sufficient to maintain functional viability of the muscle tissue. The degree of disuse atrophy can be limited by electrical stimulation.

	AXON TERMINAL	AXON	NEURON	MUSCLE
RESPONSE TO INJURY				
IMMEDIATELY	Loss of synaptic and trophic activity	Loss of transport past lesion site		
0 – 24 HRS.	Swelling	. Disruption of mitochondria . Proliferation of neurofibrils and neurofilaments . Beading of process distal to and shortly proximal to lesion site		. Shortening of secondary synaptic clefts . Widening of synaptic cleft . Decrease in receptor density at nmj.
1 – 7 DAYS	Phagocytosis	. Phagocytosis of beaded portions . Myelin sheath withdrawal	Nissl "degeneration"	. Dedifferentiation of nmj. . Increase in ACh sensitivity over entire cell . Fasciculation
7 DAYS +		Growth cone development		Decrease in number of contractile proteins
1 MONTH +		Process extension along endoneurial tube		Contraction in response to electrical stimulation
REGENERATION				
2 – 6 MONTHS	Re-establishment of axon terminal	Regrowth to neuromuscular junction	Return to normal function and staining	Re-establishment of nmj.
6 – 12 MONTHS		Remyelination		Increase in number of contractile proteins
DEGENERATION				
2 MONTHS +	Regrowth blocked anatomically or functionally		Death	Fibrosis OR Re-innervation by adjacent axon sprout

Figure 5-5. Response to somatomotor neuron process injury in the peripheral nervous system.

Review Exercises

5-1.   One of the more promising restorative techniques currently developing in neurology is normal fetal neural tissue implantation for replacement of diseased or traumatized central neural tissue. What assumptions concerning the developmental potentials of both fetal and mature neural tissue underlie the use of transplantation of such tissue for the treatment of degenerative diseases such as Parkinsonism?

5-2.   The sural nerve is the most commonly used source of experimental peripheral neural transplants into the spinal cord.
   a. Why would this be a nerve of preference? What classes of peripheral nerve fibers are in the sural nerve?
   b. Outline and diagram the expected events following sural nerve segment transplantation into the transected spinal cord. Indicate what potential advantages for spinal cord regeneration are supplied by the implanted tissue.
   c. Spinal implants such as that provided by the sural nerve still do not provide complete functional regeneration even under carefully controlled experimental conditions. Describe some essential trophic and functional barriers to functional regeneration following a transplant procedure.

5-3.   Refer to Patient #1 in the Appendix.
   a. Explain the results of the nerve conduction velocity examinations in terms of the events you would expect to see happening following a complete lesion of a peripheral nerve.
   b. Justify the use of a nerve graft for repair of the injury to the ulnar nerve. Why would the sural nerve be a reasonable choice for the source of the graft? Is it necessary that the grafted nerve contain the same types of peripheral nerve fibers as the injured nerve?
   c. Assuming that the nerve graft is effective and regeneration occurs, describe the events you would expect to see happen with healing. Consider also:

   • The length of time you would expect to have elapse before a normal conduction velocity and EMG examination would be recorded.
   • The probability that the same type and number of motor units would be found in the hypothenar muscles following regeneration of the nerve as before the injury.
   • The probability that sensory function of the ulnar side of the hand would be normal following regeneration.

5-4.   From your knowledge about the time of development of gross structures and cytoarchitecture within the central nervous system, relate the developmental abnormalities listed to the most likely time at which alteration in development or pathology could cause each abnormality.

Abnormalities
- spina bifida: incomplete closure of the neural tube in the lumbar region
- anencephaly: lack of development of the cerebral hemispheres
- spastic diplegic cerebral palsy: spasticity (hypertonus) of both lower extremities with evidence of poor myelination of the lateral corticospinal tract
- cerebellar ataxia in cerebral palsy: poor motor coordination with evidence of faulty processing of motor control information in the cerebellum
- Parkinson's disease: degeneration of previously normally functioning dopamine producing cells in the basal ganglia and other areas of the CNS

Times of disruption of development
- within the first two weeks of fetal development
- within the first two months of fetal development
- at the time of birth with full term infant
- within two days post delivery, full term infant
- within two months post delivery, full term infant
- within the first two years of life
- following maturity

6

Spinal Cord Anatomy

The spinal cord is the one portion of the CNS that largely retains at maturity its embryonic segmental nature. The spinal cord segmental nerves roughly correspond in number to the vertebral segments; thus, there are 8 cervical nerves, 12 thoracic, 5 lumbar, 5 sacral and 1 coccygeal. The eighth cervical nerve owes its presence to the first cervical nerve (which is purely sensory) that is found cranial to the first cervical vertebra. Due to the elongation of the vertebral column relative to the spinal cord during development, only the highest spinal segments correspond horizontally with the vertebral foramina through which the nerves pass. The level of correspondence is continuously changing with growth. At maturity, the spinal cord terminates at L1-L3 vertebral level in persons of normal height. The lower spinal nerves en route to their corresponding foramina form the cauda equina within the spinal canal.

In cross section, the spinal cord demonstrates a central, butterfly-shaped region of grey matter containing cell bodies, terminal axons, and short processes. The relative size and total amount of grey and white matter varies at different spinal levels. The percentage of white matter decreases descending in the cord. The volume of grey matter is greatest at the levels at which the cervical, brachial, and lumbar plexus cell bodies are located, leading to regional enlargement of the cord at these levels. These variations in volume as well as the shape of the central grey matter provide useful landmarks for identification of spinal levels in cross section.

General Organization of the Grey Matter

The grey matter represents a continuous cell column over the length of the spinal cord. Not only the cell bodies are related to body segments, but the entry and exit of segmental nerves are relatively well concentrated on a segmental basis. Looked at diagrammatically, as in Figure 6-1, segmental zones can be seen to represent areas of concentration and overlap for somatic segment innervation. The segmental relationship is considerably more diffuse for autonomic (visceral) motor control and sensation than for somatic. At any

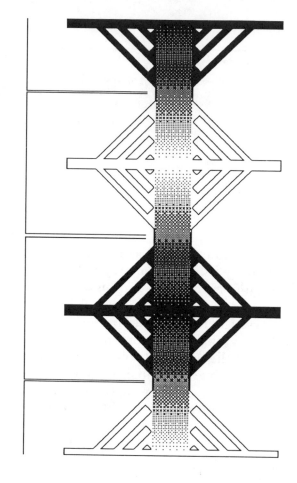

Figure 6-1. Segmental concentration of neuron cell bodies in the spinal cord. *White* areas represent neuron cell bodies and processes related to the T-8 or T-10 spinal nerves. *Black* areas represent neuron cell bodies and processes related to T-9 or T-7 spinal nerves.

given level as viewed in cross section, the grey matter shows a typical and consistent organization of cells . The basic division of cells follows the embryonic pattern, with motor cells located ventral to the sulcus limitans in the ventral and intermediolateral horns and sensory cells located in the dorsal horn. Within these basic sensory and motor divisions, cell groups with relatively specific and well-identified function are divided into lamina, as first described by Rexed, and into nuclear groups (Fig. 6-2).

Laminae I-VI form the dorsal horn. Lamina I is also termed the nucleus marginalis in some regions of the spinal cord. It serves as the termination point for small diameter sensory fibers, typically type C afferents. Laminae II-III are termed the substantia gelatinosa as a result of their vacuolar appearance in some types of histological preparations. The substantia gelatinosa also serves as a termination point for the smaller primary afferents as well as the receiving point for input both from interneurons located in more ventral laminae and from some descending spinal fibers. Parts of laminae IV and V form the nucleus proprius of the dorsal horn. This region of the dorsal horn receives direct primary afferent input from the entire range of sensory fibers,

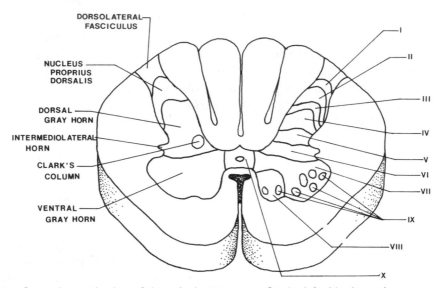

Figure 6-2. General organization of the spinal grey matter. On the left side the major groups of cell bodies are indicated. The right side shows the laminar organization.

with the possible exception of the C fibers. Cell bodies in this region have processes that may project as short interneurons or that may form long ascending spinal tracts. Clarke's nucleus is located in the medial portion of lamina VI at lumbar and thoracic levels of the cord. It also probably receives direct sensory input, primarily from large diameter fibers. Cell bodies in Clarke's nucleus send fibers into ascending spinal tracts. The named regions of the laminae described in the dorsal horn are variably present at different levels of the spinal cord; they are most evident at the lumbar and cervical enlargements.

The ventral horn contains laminae VII-X. The laminar grouping of cell bodies fairly evident at all cord levels in the dorsal horn is not clear in the ventral horn. Lamina VII borders lamina VI and penetrates a variable distance ventrally into the ventral horn. It contains interneuron cell bodies, cell bodies with projections into propriospinal and ascending spinal tracts, and cell bodies of preganglionic sympathetic and parasympathetic neurons. The sympathetic preganglionic neurons are collected laterally into the intermediolateral horn of the thoracic spinal cord. In the lumbar and sacral levels, preganglionic neuron cell bodies for sympathetic and parasympathetic neurons are located in essentially the same place in lamina VII, but as a result of the lumbar enlargement of the ventral horn, the intermediolateral horn is no longer evident. Lamina VIII contains interneuron cell bodies that receive input from the dorsal horn and propriospinal and descending spinal tracts. These interneurons in turn project onto the somatomotor neurons of lamina IX (and the preganglionic neurons of lamina VII). Laminae VIII and IX are intermixed, with cells of lamina IX forming nuclear clusters or islands within lamina VIII. The cells in lamina IX are the alpha and gamma motorneurons of the somatomotor system. In the cervical and lumbar enlargements related to innervation of the extremities, the motorneurons are grouped with the neurons for distal muscles located laterally and those for proximal muscles medially. In addition to this proximal-distal orientation, neurons for physiological flexors are located relatively dorsally, while those for physiological extensors are located ventrally.

The last lamina of the spinal grey matter is lamina X, located centrally around the residual central canal. Cells in this region are interneurons.

General Organization of the White Matter

The white matter of the spinal cord can be separated longitudinally into three major funiculi: dorsal, lateral, and ventral (Fig. 6-3). The dorsal and lateral funiculi are separated by the posterior lateral sulcus that marks the entry line of the dorsal root fibers and the tip of the dorsal horn. The division between lateral and ventral funiculi is demarcated less clearly by the exit line of the ventral rootlets. The two halves of the spinal cord are separated dorsally by the posterior median sulcus and septum and ventrally by the much more prominent anterior or ventral sulcus. At the upper thoracic and cervical levels, the dorsal funiculus is divided by the posterior intermediate sulcus into two subdivisions, or fasciculi: the lateral fasciculus gracilis and the medial fasciculus cuneatus.

The white matter contains axons that can be classed into the following major categories:

1. Long ascending axons with cell bodies in the spinal grey or dorsal root ganglia and terminations at brainstem or higher levels. These fibers have either a sensory or a system state feedback function.
2. Long descending axons with cell bodies at the brainstem level or above and terminations in the spinal grey at various levels (and laminae). These fibers have both motor control and sensory modulation functions.
3. Long and short propriospinal axons with origin and termination within the spinal cord. The cells of origin for these fibers are spinal interneurons with integrative and association functions.
4. Propriospinal axon collaterals from primary sensory afferents.
5. Commissural fibers crossing from one side of the cord to the other.

Propriospinal fibers are located in a narrow band completely surrounding the grey matter. Within this band, fibers are organized on the basis of the distance they will travel before reentering the grey matter. Longer fibers are positioned more eccentrically. Propriospinal sensory collateral axons are located near the main ascending fibers either at the tip of the dorsal horn (Lissauer's tract) or between the fasciculi gracilis and cuneatus (coma tract). Commissural fibers are found predominantly in the anterior white commissure, although some cross through lamina X. The long descending pathways are found in the lateral and ventral funiculi, and the long ascending pathways are located in

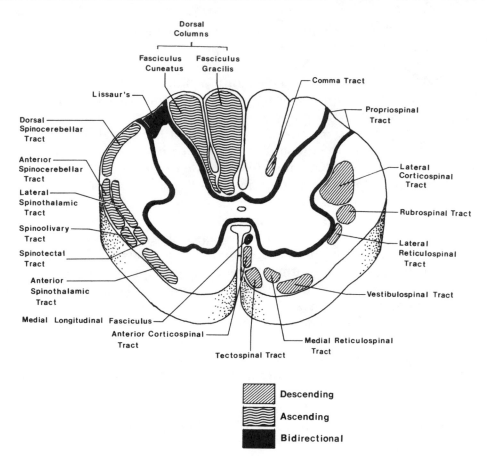

Figure 6-3. Diagrammatic representation of ascending and descending spinal white matter tracts as seen in a generalized cervical cross section.

the dorsal funiculi (dorsal columns) and along the outer margins in the lateral and ventral funiculi. Specific fiber bundles can be identified for the long pathways, but there is considerable overlap and intermingling among pathways in many cases.

Long Spinal Pathways or Tracts

The long spinal tracts of the cord are typically described in terms of the following characteristics:
1. Original identified function (motor or sensory).
2. The number of neurons in the pathway chain between origin and termination or, alternatively, the number of synapses in the pathway.
3. The location of the cells of origin of the pathway.
4. The location of major synapses in the pathway.
5. The location of the primary axon termination of the chain.
6. The level of decussation (unless the pathway remains ipsilateral).
7. The location of the fibers in the spinal white matter.

Spinal tracts (and most other CNS pathways) are named on the basis of either their origin and destination (thus "corticospinal" with the origin in the cortex and the termination in the spinal cord) or their anatomical location or appearance (thus "dorsal columns" for the major touch discriminatory tracts because of their location in the dorsal portion of the spinal cord). Tables 6-1 and 6-2 summarize the major spinal tracts.

The ascending sensory or system state tracts of the spinal cord have their cells of origin either in the dorsal root ganglia or in the interneurons of the dorsal horn. They ascend in the white matter of the spinal cord and pass through the brainstem to terminate in one of three locations: the reticular formation of the brainstem, the cerebellum, or the thalamus. Many tracts with a synapse in the thalamus project by thalamocortical neurons through the internal capsule to the somatosensory regions of the cerebral cortex. The descending motor control or sensory modulatory tracts of the spinal cord terminate in the spinal grey either 1) ventrally on alpha and gamma motor neurons or their associated interneurons, autonomic preganglionic neurons, or associated interneurons or 2) dorsally on primary afferents (presynaptically) or higher order sensory neurons. The cells of origin of descending tracts are found predominantly in the motor and sensory cortex of the cerebral hemispheres, the hypothalamus, the nuclei of cranial nerves, and the brainstem reticular formation. (Two other motor regions, the basal ganglia and the cerebellum, do not send direct projections to the spinal cord.) Fibers with their origin in the cerebral hemispheres pass through the internal capsule and the brainstem before reaching the spinal cord. The characteristics of the major spinal pathways are outlined in Tables 6-1 and 6-2. At various levels of the cord, some spinal tracts are not evident because they contain either ascending fibers that have not yet entered the cord or descending fibers that have already terminated.

Description of Specific Spinal Tracts

Ascending Tracts with Synapses in the Thalamus

Projections to the thalamus carry various sensory modalities. There are two major collections of fibers projecting to the thalamus: the dorsal columns contained in the fasciculi cuneatus and gracilis and the spinothalamic tracts (lateral and anterior or ventral) located in the lateral funiculus.

The dorsal columns (Fig. 6-4) carry epicritic (discriminatory) touch and pressure sensation and proprioceptive information (kinesthesia), and, as might be expected, contain large diameter fibers. Fibers in the dorsal columns are somatotopically organized: the fasciculus gracilis contains fibers arising from dorsal root ganglia from Coc-1 to T-4 and the fasciculus cuneatus contains fibers from T-3 through C-5 levels. Fibers carrying the same information from the upper cervical levels are contained in the accessory cuneate fasciculus. With only two synapses, the first in the gracile and cuneate nuclei of the medulla and the second in the ventral posterior lateral nucleus of the

TABLE 6-1. Major Ascending Tracts of the Spinal Cord

Name	Synapse 1°	Location 2°	Level of Decussation	Origin	Destination	Function
Dorsal Columns						
Fasciculus Gracilis	nucleus gracilis	VPL nuc. thalamus	medulla: internal arcuate fibers	DRG Co-1 to T-6	cerebral cortex; primary sensori-motor regions	discrete somatotopic transfer of touch, vibration, kinesthesia
Fasciculus Cuneatus	nucleus cuneatus	VPL nuc. thalamus	medulla: internal arcuate fibers	DRG T-5 to C-1	cerebral cortex; primary sensori-motor regions	discrete somatotopic transfer of touch, vibration, kinesthesia
Spinothalamic Tracts						
Anterior (Ventral)	laminae I, IV, V	VPL nuc. thalamus	1-2 segments above level of entry	laminae I, IV, V	· thalamus · brainstem periaque-ductal grey	somatotopic transfer of affective light touch, pain, temperature
Lateral	laminae I, IV, V	VPL nuc. thalamus	1-2 segments above level of entry	laminae I, IV, V	· thalamus · brainstem reticular formation	somatotopic transfer of affective light touch, pain, temperature
Spinocerebellar Tracts						
Ventral (Anterior)	base of dorsal horn		· level of entry · superior cerebellar peduncle	dorsal horn	cerebellum	somatotopic transfer of proprioception
Dorsal (Posterior)	Clarke's nucleus			L-3 to C-8	cerebellum	somatotopic transfer of spinal interneuron activity
Cuneocerebellar	accessory cuneate nucleus			C-7 to C-2	cerebellum	somatotopic transfer of spinal interneuron activity
Spinobrainstem Tracts						
Spinoreticular	dorsal horn		bilateral	dorsal horn	brainstem reticular formation	nondiscrim-inative transfer of touch, pro-prioception
Spinotectal	dorsal horn		· level of entry · brainstem	dorsal horn	superior colliculus	nondiscrim-inative transfer of touch, pro-prioception
Spino-Olivary	dorsal horn		bilateral		inferior olivary nucleus	somatotopic transfer of spinal interneuron activity

TABLE 6-2. Major Descending Tracts of the Spinal Cord

Name	Origin	Destination	Decussation	Function
Corticospinal Tracts				
Lateral Corticospinal	primary motor and sensory cortex	· laminae VIII, IX · dorsal horn	medulla: decussation of the pyramids	· control alpha, gamma motor neurons · modulate 1° afferents
Anterior Corticospinal	· primary and secondary motor cortex · sensory cortex	· laminae VIII, IX · dorsal horn	ipsilateral	· control alpha, gamma motor neurons · modulate 1° afferents
Rubrospinal Tract	red nucleus	· laminae VIII, IX · dorsal horn	midbrain	· control alpha, gamma motor neurons · modulate 1° afferents
Tectospinal Tract	superior colliculus	· laminae VIII, IX cervical levels	midbrain	· control alpha, gamma motor neurons
Vestibulospinal Tracts				
Lateral Vestibulospinal	Deiter's nucleus	· laminae VIII, IX	bilateral	· control alpha, gamma motor neurons
Medial Longitudinal Fasciculus (MLF)	vestibular nuclei	laminae VIII, IX cervical levels	bilateral	· control alpha, gamma motor neurons
Reticulospinal Tracts				
Somatomotor	reticular formation	laminae VIII, IX	bilateral	· control alpha, gamma motor neurons
Autonomic	reticular formation	lamina VII: thoracic and lumbo-sacral levels	bilateral	· control autonomic preganglionic neurons
Sensory	· raphe nuclei · reticular formation	dorsal horn	bilateral	· modulate 1° afferents

thalamus, the dorsal columns are well suited for rapid delivery of epicritic sensation to the primary sensory and motor cortex.

The spinothalamic tracts (Fig. 6-5) carry sensory information concerning temperature, light or protopathic touch, and pain. The cell bodies for both spinothalamic tracts are located in various laminae of the dorsal horn, primarily lamina I for pain sensation and lamina V for temperature, touch, and some additional pain submodalities. Projections in the lateral spinothalamic tract to the ventral posterior lateral nucleus of the thalamus are somatotopically organized and represent a fairly specific location coded transfer of informa-

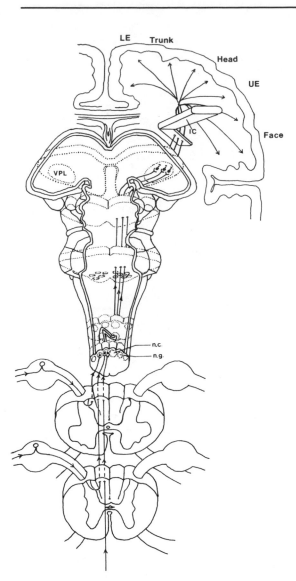

Figure 6-4. Dorsal columns. The pathways used are, from spinal to cortical, the fasciculi gracilis and cuneatus in the spinal cord, the medial lemniscus in the brainstem, the internal capsule in the diencephalon and the corona radiata in the cerebral hemispheres. Note the somatotopic projection. *IC,* internal capsule; *LE,* lower extremity; *n.c.,* nucleus cuneatus; *n.g.,* nucleus gracilis; *UE,* upper extremity; *VPL,* ventral posterior lateral nucleus of the thalamus.

tion. The anterior spinothalamic tract differs by having convergent input to many of its neurons of origin, with convergence of both modality and location information. Its information thus is much more generalized. Both spinothalamic pathways, but probably predominantly the anterior one, send collateral projections into the reticular formation of the brainstem. Fibers in the spinothalamic tracts vary in diameter from fairly large to very small; there appears to be a close correlation between the size of the relevant primary afferent fiber and the size of the ascending fiber.

Ascending Tracts with Termination in the Cerebellum

There are three main projections to the cerebellum: the anterior (ventral)

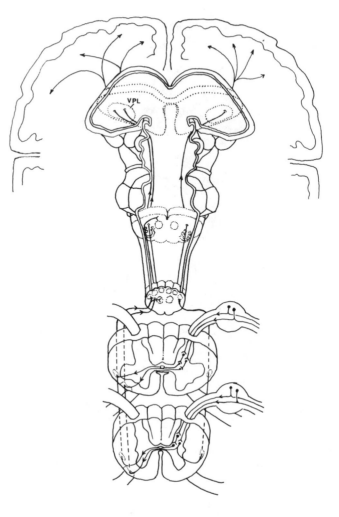

Figure 6-5. Spinothalamic tracts. The decussating fibers in the spinal cord complete their cross within one to two segments above the level of entry of the primary afferent fibers. The lateral spinothalamic tract is shown projecting bilaterally. Although termed the spinothalamic tract, information carried in this pathway is projected from the thalamus to the sensory cortex in a somatotopic fashion similar to that seen for the information carried in the dorsal columns. *VPL,* ventral posterior lateral nucleus of thalamus.

and posterior (dorsal) spinocerebellar tracts and the cuneocerebellar tract (Figs. 6-6, 6-7). All of these pathways carry information used by the cerebellum in determining commands for motor control. The posterior spinocerebellar and cuneocerebellar tracts carry somatotopically organized information from proprioceptors of various kinds. The posterior spinocerebellar tract has its cells of origin in Clarke's nucleus; the cuneocerebellar tract carries information from cervical levels and has cells of origin in the accessory cuneate nucleus of the dorsal horn. The anterior spinocerebellar tract has cells of origin in the base of the dorsal horn (laminae IV, V, and VI) and possibly also from motor interneurons in lamina VII and VIII; it carries predominantly system state feedback information. This information essentially is a report to the cerebellum of the state of activity in spinal interneuronal motor networks. Both types of spinocerebellar tracts allow for very rapid delivery of information to the cerebellum. The posterior spinocerebellar and cuneocerebellar tracts, in particular, are made up of large diameter fibers and transmit

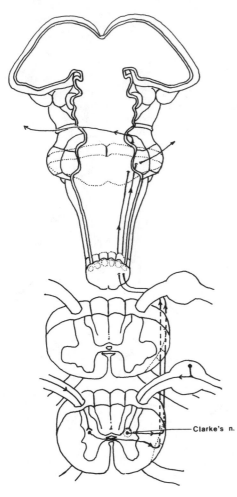

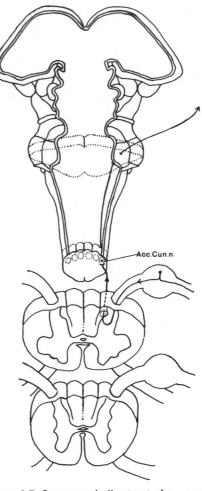

Figure 6-6. Anterior (ventral) and posterior (dorsal) spinocerebellar tracts. As is typical of projection to and from the cerebellum, information relating to one side of the body is dealt with in the same side of the cerebellum. This requires that spinal tracts either do not decussate (as is true for the posterior spinocerebellar tract) or decussate twice (as for the anterior spinocerebellar tract). The second decussation of this tract occurs within the superior cerebellar peduncle and the white matter of the cerebellum.

Figure 6-7. Cuneocerebellar tract. *Acc., cun. n.,* accessory cuneate nucleus.

information with only one synapse in the spinal cord before it is sent directly to the cerebellar cortex.

Ascending Tracts with Termination in the Brainstem

Many of the nuclear groups of the brainstem and the reticular formation receive input from the spinal cord (Fig. 6-8). Transmission of information in these pathways may be organized somatotopically to a certain extent. There

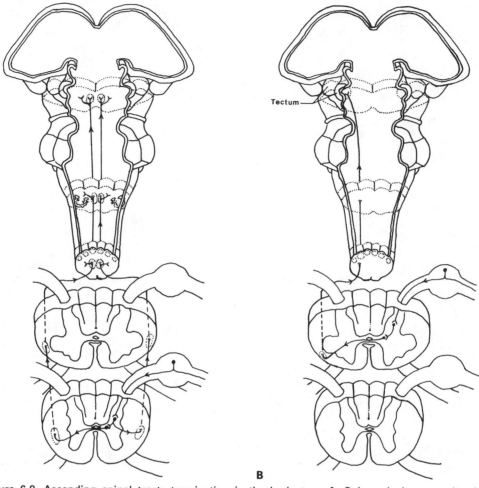

A   **B**

Figure 6-8. Ascending spinal tracts terminating in the brainstem. **A.** Spinoreticular tract showing bilateral projection of information with distribution into the reticular formation at all brainstem levels. **B.** Spinotectal track showing predominantly contralateral projection to the tectum of the midbrain, primarily the superior colliculus.

appears to be a strong correlation between the types of activity controlled by various brainstem structures and the type of sensory information projected to them. As examples, the spinotectal tract carries somatotopically organized touch and proprioceptive information useful for informing the tectum of the brainstem about the position of the body. The spino-olivary tract also carries information about body position and movement. A great deal of this information, like that carried in the anterior spinocerebellar tract, deals with the state of excitation and the type of activity occuring in spinal motor interneuron networks. The spinoreticular tract carries nondiscriminative touch, pain, and temperature information from various parts of the body to specific regions of the reticular formation. Sensory information from internal organs is an important part of the information carried in this pathway. Speed of transmission

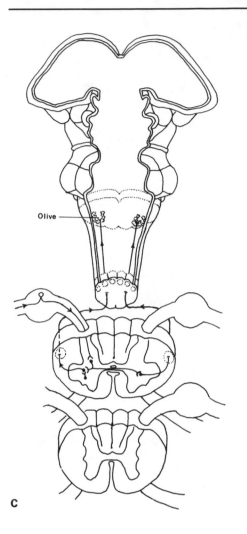

Olive

Figure 6-8.
C. Spino-olivary tract showing bilateral projection to the
inferior olivary nucleus of
the medulla.

c

in spinobrainstem pathways is quite variable. Fiber diameter covers a wide range. Classically, these tracts were thought to be entirely multisynaptic, but now many projections are recognized to by monosynaptic or disynaptic.

Descending Tracts Originating in the Cerebral Cortex

The anterior and lateral corticospinal tracts originate in the motor regions of the frontal lobe and the primary sensory regions of the parietal lobe and descend through the internal capsule to enter the ventral surface of the brainstem in the cerebral peduncles (Fig. 6-9). These tracts continue in a dispersed form through the pons and then form the pyramids on the ventral surface of the medulla (hence the name "pyramidal" tract). Fibers forming the lateral corticospinal tract, approximately 90% of the pyramidal fibers, cross in the decussation of the pyramids in the medulla. In the spinal cord, the lateral corticospinal tract lies near the dorsal horn in the lateral funiculus. The remaining pyramidal fibers descend ipsilaterally in the ventral funiculus of

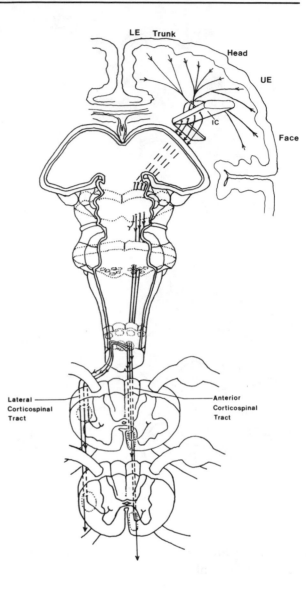

Figure 6-9. Corticospinal tracts. Descending pathways involve the corona radiata, internal capsule *(IC)* in the diencephalon, cerebral peduncles in the midbrain, pyramids in the medulla, and the anterior (ipsilateral) and lateral (contralateral) corticospinal tracts in the spinal cord. Note the somatotopic origin of the tract in the frontal lobe.

the spinal cord, forming the anterior corticospinal tract. Sensory modulation fibers found primarily in the lateral corticospinal tract terminate within various laminae of the dorsal horn. Their contacts are either presynaptic on primary afferent fibers or postsynaptic on sensory interneurons or sensory fibers projecting into ascending spinal tracts. Motor control fibers from both lateral and anterior corticospinal tracts terminate, without prior synapses, either on motor interneurons in lamina VIII or directly on alpha and gamma motorneurons in lamina IX of the ventral horn. The anterior corticospinal tract primarily innervates motor neurons or interneurons related to trunk muscles; the lateral tract predominantly innervates proximal and distal extremity muscles. The lateral corticospinal tract has the distinction of containing some neurons with large cell bodies (Betz cells) in the primary motor cortex and terminations directly on alpha motor neurons. Throughout their length, the corticospinal tract fibers are somatotopically organized.

Descending Tracts Originating in the Brainstem

Generally speaking, descending brainstem tracts are reciprocal with ascending tracts terminating in the brainstem. From cranial to caudal, there is the tectospinal tract, the rubrospinal tract, two vestibulospinal tracts, and a collection of reticulospinal fibers (Figs. 16-10 through 16-13). The tectospinal tract originates in the superior colliculus of the midbrain, decussates within the midbrain, and descends to terminate on motor neurons and interneurons predominantly at cervical levels. The rubrospinal tract originates in the red nucleus of the midbrain and immediately decussates. It descends in close

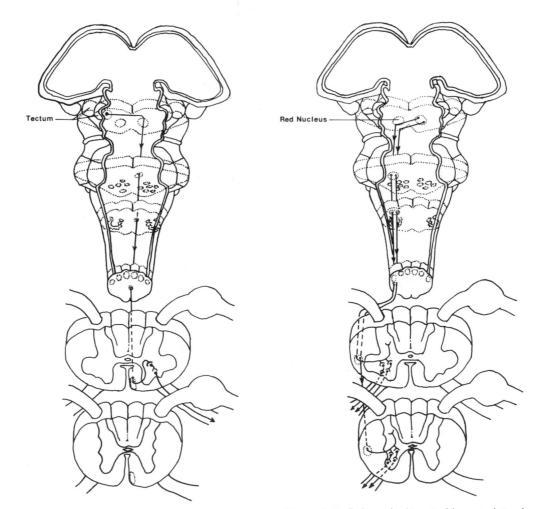

Figure 6-10. Tectospinal tract. This tract projects visual information contralaterally to the spinal cord, primarily to cervical levels.

Figure 6-11. Rubrospinal tract with contralateral projection to the spinal cord.

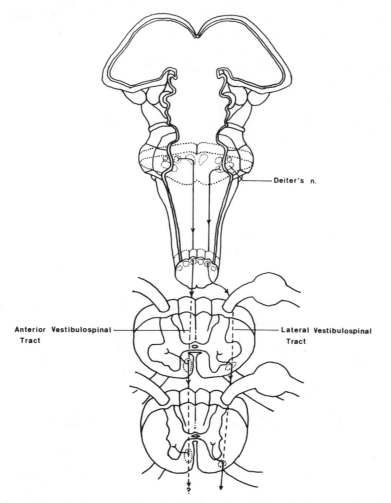

Figure 6-12. Vestibulospinal tracts. Fibers in the lateral vestibulospinal tract arise primarily from Deiter's nucleus (lateral vestibular nucleus). Fibers in the anterior vestibulospinal tract or spinal portion of the medial longitudinal fasciculus arise from all vestibular nuclei.

relationship to the lateral corticospinal tract in the lateral funiculus of the cord. It terminates on motor neurons or interneurons, primarily ones that control movement of trunk and proximal limb muscles. The vestibulospinal tracts originate in the nuclei of the vestibular nerve in the caudal pons. Projections are both ipsilateral and contralateral. The ventral (anterior) vestibulospinal tract terminates on motor neurons and interneurons controlling neck and possibly trunk muscles. The lateral vestibulospinal tract extends the length of the cord and controls both trunk and proximal extremity muscles.

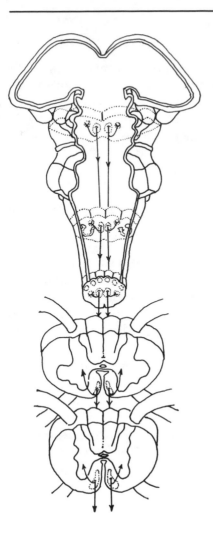

Figure 6-13. Reticulospinal tracts. These multiple pathways carry somatomotor, sensory modulation and autonomic motor information bilaterally from all levels of the brainstem reticular formation to their appropriate termination in the spinal cord.

Through connections with the cerebellum, the vestibulospinal tracts (and possibly to a minor extent the rubrospinal tract) provide a means of transmitting motor control information from the cerebellum to the spinal cord. The cerebellum itself has no direct projection to the spinal cord. Reticulospinal fibers carry both somatomotor and autonomic motor information in addition to sensory modulatory information, from various brainstem reticular locations. Reticulospinal projects may be contralateral, but they are predominantly ipsilateral.

Review Exercises

6-1.   The location and extent of spinal cord lesions can be estimated clinically by testing for the presence of conscious awareness, discrimination and localization of specific sensory stimuli and by testing for the presence of motor control of muscles innervated from each level of the cord. What deficits in sensory and motor function would you expect to see as a result of each of the lesions of the spinal cord listed below? In each case consider:

- sensory modalities lost (what tracts are involved)
- motor control lost

a. Hemisection (loss of all of the right or left half of the cord) at any spinal level. This deficit leads to what is clinically termed a Brown-Sequard syndrome.

b Degeneration in the mid-cervical levels (C3-C6) of the central material of the spinal cord involving all of laminae III-VI and X, most of lamina VII, and centrally-located portions of laminae I, II and XI. Inner portions of the white matter in the dorsal and lateral funiculi are typically also involved. This type of a lesion occurs with pathological expansion of the central canal such as is found in syringomyelia.

c. Selective dorsal rhizotomy (section of the dorsal root or rootlets between the dorsal root ganglia and the cord) over segments L1-L3 unilaterally. This type of a surgical lesion was performed historically to manage intractable pain, and is currently being used to manage persistent muscle hypertonia (spasticity) in children with cerebral palsy. In addition to considering the questions raised above concerning tracts involved, discuss possible explanations for the frequent observation that chronic pain recurred several months following dorsal rhizotomy, even when there was no evidence of dorsal root regeneration.

6-2.   Structural Models

Three-dimensional realization of the central nervous system is typically difficult to generate when only sectional views are available. A number of modeling projects can assist in developing a sense of relative location of CNS structures of major importance. Although computer-generated three-dimensional representations of the CNS have been produced, they are not yet widely available, and they do not permit tactile learning of spatial relationships. To review the material in Chapter 6, the following models are suggested:

1. Spinal cross sections. Prepare a cross section of the spinal cord at any general level (cervical, thoracic, lumbar) and show on the section the location of the grey matter laminae and the white matter tracts, differentiating ascending, descending and bidirectional tracts.

2. Spinal tracts. Prepare several cross-sections of the spinal cord and connect them with selected spinal tracts. Use this type of a model to demonstrate relative tract position and decussation of fibers leading into or actually in the tracts.

7

Spinal Sensorimotor Integration

Within the spinal cord, sensory (primary afferent) neurons, interneurons, and motor (efferent) neurons are organized into functional networks that permit elementary integration of sensory information and motor behavior. The same basic potential for sensorimotor integration can be seen at the brainstem level involving the cranial nerves and is used as a basic model for the development of more complex sensorimotor integration networks involving higher levels of the neuraxis.

There are four essential components of any reflex arc (Fig. 7-1):

1. A sensory receptor.
2. A primary afferent neuron.
3. A motor neuron.
4. An effector.

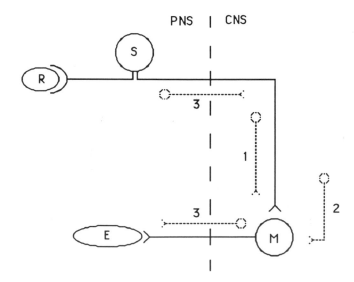

Figure 7-1. Components of a relfex arc. *E,* effector; *I,* integration neuron; *M,* motor neuron; *R,* sensory receptor; *S,* sensory neuron. In any reflex system additional complexity may occur through multiplication of the integrator system (1), additional central input to the motor neuron (2), and multiplication of the sensory and motor components (3).

These basic components in any spatially extended system will be connected by afferent and efferent lines of communication (sensory and motor nerve fibers).

The basic reflex arc may be modified in any one of the following ways:
1. Interposition of one or more interneurons between the afferent and efferent cells.
2. Modification of sensory or motor cell activity through input to the arc from other CNS regions.
3. Increase in the number and complexity of interrelationships of the sensory or motor cells involved.

The spinal reflex pathways that have been studied in most detail and with which this chapter is primarily concerned involve the somatomotor system. Autonomic reflexes also exist within the spinal cord and almost certainly are organized very much like somatomotor reflexes.

Alpha and gamma motor neurons can be classed in the following categories:
1. Homonymous motor neurons: innervate the muscle from which the relevant stimulus arises.
2. Synergist motor neurons: innervate muscles that have similar or supportive functions to the one(s) from which the stimulus arises. These motor neurons either may relate only to muscles acting at one joint, or they may be grouped functionally into muscles that act together at several adjacent joints, such as limb flexor muscles.
3. Antagonist motor neurons: innervate muscle(s) with actions contrary to those from which the stimulus arises.
4. Ipsilateral motor neurons: located on the same side of the spinal cord as the incoming sensory information.
5. Contralateral motor neurons: located on the opposite side of the spinal cord from the incoming sensory information.

Alpha and Gamma Activation

In most cases, alpha and gamma motor neurons to the same muscle are activated concurrently, or coactivated. This is not the same thing as cocontraction of agonist-antagonist muscle groups acting on the same joint. Because of the variety of types of both alpha and gamma motor neurons to any one muscle, coactivation can produce an extremely wide range of muscle behavior, depending on the exact pattern of coactivation used. The decision of which type of gamma motor neuron to activate is dependent on the desired quality of muscle contraction, as described earlier. There is still much investigation to be done concerning the type of gamma activation occurring in various spinal reflexes. The basic networks that permit flexible use of alpha and gamma motor neurons is laid down, or "hardwired," in the spinal sensorimotor reflexes. These networks can then be used in a flexible way by descending motor control pathways.

The basic spinal reflexes include the following:
1. Monosynaptic stretch reflex (myotatic reflex, deep tendon reflex).
2. Ib inhibitory reflex (inverse myotatic reflex).
3. Flexor reflex afferent reflexes (FRAs).

Monosynaptic Reflex

The monosynaptic stretch reflex is the simplest reflex in the human. Its essential components are the basic four of a reflex arc (Fig. 7-2). The receptor is the muscle spindle, the afferent neuron is the Ia fiber from the spindle primary endings, the efferent neuron is the homonymous alpha motor neuron (innervating the muscle fibers in the motor unit most closely adjacent to the activated spindle), and the effector is the extrafusal fibers of that motor unit. The central control unit for the system consists of the cell bodies of all relevant alpha motor neurons. The reflex is an example of negative feedback control. In its least complicated form, the monosynaptic stretch reflex does not involve coactivation of alpha and gamma motor neurons; it is the only existing somatomotor reflex pathway with this distinction. At least one additional component is added to this reflex pathway to make it functionally more effective. A collateral branch from the primary Ia fiber communicates with an inhibitory interneuron (the so-called "Ia inhibitory interneuron," which has been anatomically and physiologically identified). This inhibitory interneuron in turn communicates with the antagonist alpha motor neuron pool. By this means, excitation and contraction of the homonymous agonist muscle is coupled securely with inhibition of the alpha motor neurons to, and therefore relaxation of, the antagonist muscle. Complementary stretch reflex networks exist between all known agonist-antagonist motor neuron pairs. The Ia afferent also sends collateral branches to a variety of other destinations (divergent

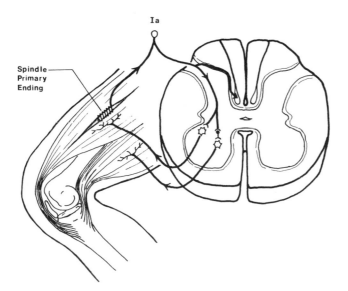

Figure 7-2. Anatomical substrate for the monosynaptic stretch reflex. The Ia afferent from the muscle spindle makes excitatory contact with the homonymous alpha motor neuron pool, the Ia inhibitory interneuron, and other sets of motor and interneurons at other spinal levels through projections in the coma tract. The Ia inhibitory interneuron acts on the antagonist alpha motor neuron pool.

pathways), some of which are at higher levels of the neuraxis such as the cerebellum and the somatosensory cortex, and some of which are nearby in the spinal cord. Given a sufficiently intense stimulus, the propriospinal pathways will cause excitation of additional homonymous motor neurons and even of synergist motor neurons. In all cases, there is no alpha-gamma coactivation. Physiologically, this network is probably used to adjust muscle tension in the face of small perturbations of the controlled joint such as might occur during a sustained contraction for the purposes of maintaining posture. In these conditions, the absence of gamma motor neuron involvement in the reflex would permit small corrective alterations in muscle activity, without affecting the general control of muscle behavior or muscle stiffness. Clinically, this reflex pathway is used both in evaluation of the level of excitation of a given pool of alpha motor neurons and in treatment aimed at altering their level of excitation. Because of the lack of coactivation in this spinal pathway, any change in gamma activity observed clinically must be due to long loop (supraspinal) responses involving Ia fiber projections.

Evaluation of the state of excitation in the components of the stretch reflex arc is done either with a natural stretch stimulus, as when testing deep tendon reflexes with a reflex hammer, or with an artificial electrical stimulus, as when testing "H" (Hoffmann) reflexes. Although both of these methods activate essentially the same reflex system, there are differences between them. The natural quick stretch stimulus activates all relevant receptors and their primary afferents, including not only the spindle primary endings but also the secondary endings and the Golgi tendon organs. The motor response observed is the integrated response to all of this sensory information; to the naked eye observer, the only component active is the Ia stretch reflex. The H reflex, on the other hand, involves isolated activation of Ia fibers with a single electrical stimulus. Additional primary afferent activity that would normally occur in a stretch reflex is not present, and the response observed is elicited only by Ia synaptic activity. For general purpose evaluations, either stimulus may be used, but when detailed information is required, the evaluator must be aware of the very real differences in spinal cord activation brought about by the two stimuli.

The stretch reflex is used in treatment to elicit muscle activity and to enhance it when it is already present. The stimulus used is either a single quick manual stretch of the muscle or vibration of the muscle or its tendon. Vibration provides repeated quick stretches of small amplitude, which is a stimulus somewhat similar to the small perturbations that occur during postural activity of the muscle. The response to vibration is a tonic, or sustained, activation of the homonymous (and occasionally synergist) muscle. Additional proprioceptive stimuli are used in treatment, some of which activate the monosynaptic stretch reflex pathways; however, the activation usually is not in isolation.

Inverse Myotatic Reflex

The Ib inhibitory network supplying the substrate for the inverse myotatic reflex is only slightly more complex than the monosynaptic stretch reflex network (Fig. 7-3). The receptor is the Golgi tendon organ, and the afferent neuron is the Ib fiber. The efferent neurons are the homonymous alpha and gamma motor neurons, and the effectors are the homonymous extrafusal and intrafusal fibers. The central control unit is made up of all relevant alpha and gamma motor neuron cell bodies. In addition, there is an inhibitory interneuron (the Ib inhibitory interneuron) interposed between the Ib fiber and the homonymous motor neurons. The degree to which static versus dynamic gamma motor neurons are affected by Ib interneuron inhibition is not yet known. Activation of this pathway by application of tension to the tendon brings about motor neuron inhibition and muscle relaxation. Like the Ia reflex, the Ib system illustrates negative feedback. Increased tension on the tendon activates the system that responds with muscle relaxation, returning the tension to the level existing prior to the disturbance. Similarly to the monosynaptic stretch reflex network, collaterals from the Ib afferent innervate additional interneurons that, in this case, have an excitatory effect on the antagonist motor neurons with which they have synapses. Additional divergent collaterals transmit Ib information to higher levels of the neuraxis and to closely related synergist motor neurons within the spinal cord.

The Ib pathway cannot be used in isolation under clinical circumstances for either evaluation or treatment, for two reasons: 1) natural stimuli sufficient to excite this pathway will also be excitatory to other pathways, among them the monosynaptic stretch reflex pathway; and 2) the Ib afferent cannot be excited in isolation by electrical stimulation. Certain stimuli, such as sustained stretch on a muscle lengthened beyond its resting length (L_o), tend to activate Ib pathways more than Ia pathways, leading to decreased homonymous alpha motor neuron excitation and muscle relaxation. Although under such circumstances the Ib reflex develops much more slowly than the Ia reflex, the response decays fairly rapidly. This would suggest that the predominant

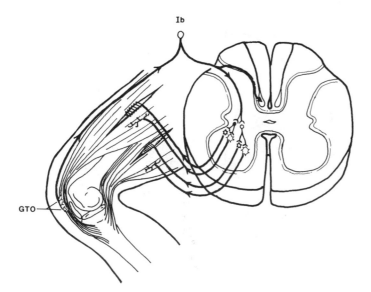

Figure 7-3. Anatomical substrate for the inverse myotatic reflex. The Ib afferent from the Golgi tendon organ (GTO) makes excitatory contact with the Ib inhibitory interneuron and with excitatory interneurons synapsing with the alpha and gamma motor neurons to the antagonist muscles. The Ib afferent also projects through the coma tract. Ib projections affect both alpha and gamma neurons.

immediate effect of Ib activation is on alpha rather than gamma motor neuron excitation. Physiologically, the Ib pathway almost certainly is used in conjunction with the Ia pathway as a means of regulating muscle stiffness as desired for various types of motor behavior. It should be obvious that because similar stimuli can elicit activity in two functionally antagonistic pathways, there must exist at the spinal level the ability to integrate information from the two to produce a response. The only cell the two pathways have in common that can serve this integrative function is the homonymous alpha motor neuron, which thus acts not only as the efferent neuron but also as the integrator of information. In the intact nervous system, modification of the effect of either the Ia fiber or the Ib fiber on the alpha motor neuron can occur through additional synapses either presynaptically on the Ia or Ib fiber or postsynaptically on the Ib interneuron. These synaptic inputs may be derived from other sensory afferents or from other regions of the CNS, which are primarily motor control pathways from higher levels of the neuraxis.

Flexor Reflex Afferent Reflexes

The flexor reflex afferent (FRA) pathway is more complex than either of the other two already discussed in that it involves chains of interneurons between the primary afferent and the motor neuron, and it routinely projects contralaterally and ipsilaterally (Fig. 7-4). A number of different stimuli can activate this pathway, including nonnoxious cutaneous stimulation, stimulation of joint receptors with group III afferents, spindle secondary receptors,

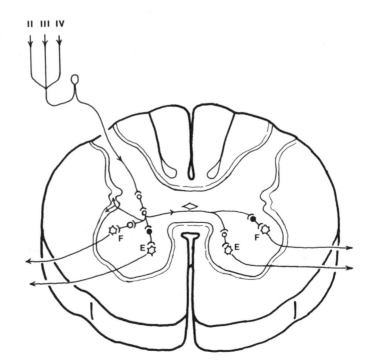

Figure 7-4. Anatomical substrate for the flexor reflex afferent response. Group II, III and IV afferents from a variety of sensory receptors project into this system. The primary branching point in the flexor reflex system is the second order interneuron. Ipsilaterally this neuron projects through an excitatory interneuron to flexor muscles (F) and through an inhibitory interneuron to extensor muscles (E). A commissural projection provides opposite control contralaterally. Projections in the propriospinal tract in both directions spread the flexor response to adjacent and distant spinal segments.

II III IV

and group III muscle afferents. The general response to appropriate stimulation of these receptors is flexion of the entire ipsilateral extremity and extension of the contralateral extremity. This full response may not always be present, depending on the modality and intensity of the stimulus and on the level of excitation of relevant alpha motor neurons. In the upper extremity in humans, the contralateral extension response is not frequently evident. Ipsilaterally, a three neuron divergent interneuron chain is interposed between the afferent neuron and the motor neuron pool. The final interneuron in one branch of this chain is excitatory to flexor motor neurons. In the other branch, the final interneuron is inhibitory to extensor motor neurons. The branch point in the chain is at the level of the second interneuron. This interneuron also sends collaterals to 1) corresponding interneuron chains on the contralateral side of the cord at the same level and 2) related motor neuron pools ipsilaterally and contralaterally at other levels of the cord, for control of other joints in the extremities. On the contralateral side of the cord, the arrangement of excitation and inhibition onto alpha motor neurons is just opposite to that on the ipsilateral side: extensors are excited and flexors are inhibited. The terminal inhibitory neuron on either side of the cord may very well be the one identified as the Ib inhibitory interneuron, illustrating the multiple use of the same anatomical substrate for different functional purposes. The inhibitory interneuron in the Ia pathway may also be involved in some cases, but its use is less likely because it does not provide alpha-gamma coactivation. Under normal circumstances, the spinal substrate of the FRA pathway may be used for a number of behaviors including flexor withdrawal, lower and upper extremity placing responses, tactile orienting responses for grasp, and gait. In gait, for example, the triggering stimulus for initiation of the flexion pattern as seen in spinal animals is ipsilateral hip extension. The relevant sensors would appear to be joint receptors.

The FRA pathway may be used clinically in treatment to elicit basic movements involving entire extremities. Due to the variety of stimuli that can elicit activity in this pathway and the divergence of information from the primary afferents involved, this reflex activity cannot always be elicited successfully. There is very definite input to the pathway at the level of the second interneuron from higher motor control centers of the neuraxis; this input can greatly modify the ability of the pathway to respond to sensory input.

Renshaw Cells

Recurrent inhibition by the Renshaw cell pathway may serve to control alpha motor neuron activity. Renshaw cells are inhibitory interneurons in lamina VIII. A given Renshaw cell is excited by a single alpha motor neuron collateral and in turn diverges to provide inhibitory synapses to the neuron of origin, homonymous neurons, and synergist alpha motor neurons. This diverging inhibitory activity may serve both to stabilize the activity of the relevant motor neurons, thereby limiting the frequency at which they can generate action potentials, and to limit the amount of synchronization within a homonymous motor neuron pool. Additional divergent projections onto antagonist alpha motor neurons may inhibit these motor neurons more than the homonymous neurons as a result of more secure synapses, thus assisting in focussing activation on the currently working pool of motor neurons.

Muscle Tone

The reflex pathways just discussed and the descending motor control pathways to be studied later all have the effect of modifying the excitability of alpha motor neurons. Essentially, they modify the resting membrane potential of the neuron and thus its probability of generating an action potential in response to any particular excitatory synaptic transmission. The Ib and FRA reflexes also directly affect gamma motor neuron activity, which in turn can alter alpha motor neuron excitability through the muscle stiffness control system. The statistical probability of alpha motor neuron response to any particular input is what is evaluated clinically as "tone". The evaluation of tone is an extremely complex process, because tone itself, and muscle stiffness, is not a standard, unvarying characteristic of alpha motor neurons. Alterations in tonic states appear to be dependent primarily on alterations in the ongoing activity in descending pathways, usually through synapses on interneurons that in turn contact the alpha and gamma motor neurons. Alterations in sensory input to spinal pathways, either under normal circumstances or in the presence of neural pathology, serve to alter motor behavior but not directly to cause long-term changes in alpha motor neuron excitability.

Review Exercises

7-1.   A Babinski reflex test is performed by firmly (but not painfully) running a sharp or rough object along the lateral ventral surface of the foot and across the ball of the foot to the base of the great toe. The normal mature response to this stimulus is flexion of the great toe. In a normal full-term infant, an adult with a spinal cord lesion at the T11-T12 level, and a person with multiple sclerosis, the Babinski reflex gives the opposite response—toe extension. Identify which spinal tract appears to be involved in producing the normal reflex response and discuss why the response would not be the normal mature response in each situation.

7-2.   Refer to Patient #4 in Appendix. Spinal Cord Injury
a. What response would you expect to see to the appropriate stimulus for the monosynaptic stretch reflex, the inverse myotatic reflex and the flexor reflex if the stimulus was delivered to afferents entering at the level of injury on the right side? On the left side? Identify what components of the three basic reflex arcs described in this chapter are affected at the level(s) of the lesion and at levels above and below the lesion.

7-3.   Functional Models

Electrical models or computer simulations may be made of the reflexes presented in this chapter integrating neural network concepts presented earlier:

1. Basic spinal reflexes (1a, 1b and FRA).
2. Long loop stretch reflexes.
3. Basic neural circuits, including inhibitory and cyclic circuits, of various types as discussed in Chapter 2.
4. Presynaptic inhibition and disinhibition (facilitation).
5. Postsynaptic summation of excitatory and inhibitory potentials.

8

Brainstem Anatomy

The basic anatomical and functional components found in the spinal cord can also be identified in the brainstem, and provides a useful and somewhat familiar framework for organizing additional brainstem structures. The main landmark components also found in the spinal cord are listed in Table 8-1. Like the spinal cord, the brainstem can be viewed as a longitudinal continuum of cell columns and fiber tracts; however, it has increased anatomical (and functional) specialization in each of its three rostrocaudal divisions: midbrain, pons, and medulla. Major fiber tracts extending the length of the brainstem or having an origin or termination within it can serve as useful landmarks even though most of them do not maintain a constant position in cross section at various levels, because of the addition or removal of tracts or the interposition of various brainstem nuclei (Tab. 8-2).

The additional anatomical and functional complexity of the brainstem arises from either the greater extent of these familiar systems (as in the reticular formation) or the addition of functions and structures unique to the brain stem. These latter additions can be grouped into the following three major categories of nuclei and associated pathways:

1. Special sensory systems (auditory, vestibular, and taste sensation).
2. Special (as opposed to general) skeletal motor control system (branchiomeric system).
3. Motor integration cells of the red nucleus, inferior olivary complex, pontine nuclei, and substantia nigra, and their connecting and projecting pathways.

TABLE 8-1. Common Landmarks: Spinal Cord and Brainstem

Grey matter	White matter
· somatomotor cell columns · visceral motor (autonomic) cell columns · visceral sensory cell columns · reticular formation (homologous to spinal interneurons)	· medial lemniscus (continuation of the dorsal column pathways) · spinothalamic tract · corticospinal (and corticobulbar) tract

TABLE 8-2. Major Brainstem Fiber Tracts and Their Function

Tract	Function	Origin	Termination
Ascending:			
*Medial Lemniscus	discriminatory sensation; body	n. gracilis, n. cuneatus	thalamus (VPL)
	discriminatory sensation; face	main sensory n. V	thalamus(VPM)
*Spinothalamic Tract	pain and temperature; body	spinal cord dorsal horn	thalamus (VPL)
Trigeminothalamic Tract	pain and temperature; face	spinal nucleus V	thalamus(VPM)
*Lateral Lemniscus	auditory sensation	cochlear nuclei	inferior colliculus
Spinocerebellar Tract			
Dorsal	proprioception	Clarke's nucleus	cerebellum (inf. ped.)
Ventral	proprioception, system state information	lateral dorsal horn	cerebellum (sup. ped.)
Descending			
*Corticospinal Tract	voluntary motor control and sensory modulation	cerebral cortex areas 6, 4, 3, 1, 2, 5	spinal cord; dorsal and ventral horn
Rubrospinal Tract	motor control	red nucleus	spinal cord
Vestibulospinal Tract	motor control	lateral vest. n.	spinal cord
Bidirectional			
*Medial Longitudinal Fasciculus	vestibular-ocular integration	vestibular and abducens nuclei	abducens, trochlear and oculomotor nuclei
	vestibular-neck integration	vestibular nuclei	cervical spinal cord
Central Tegmental Tract	reticular system-hypothalamus integration	pontine and midbrain reticular system	hypothalamus
Dorsal Longitudinal Fasciculus	reticular system-hypothalamus integration	pontine and midbrain reticular system	hypothalamus

*Readily identifiable pathways useful as landmarks.

Major External Landmarks of the Brainstem

With the cerebellum and cerebral hemispheres removed, the three divisions of the brainstem can be identified by a few major external landmarks visible from either the dorsal or the ventral view.

Dorsal Landmarks (Fig. 8-1)

The caudal extent of the medulla is delimited by the paired gracile tubercles overlying the nucleus gracilis. The cuneate tubercles are located just cranially and laterally. The fourth ventricle overlies much of the medulla; its posterior extent is the obex, positioned between the gracile tubercles. In the caudal floor of the fourth ventricle can be seen the medially placed paired hypoglossal trigones (hypoglossal nuclei), which extend cranially to the rostral limit of

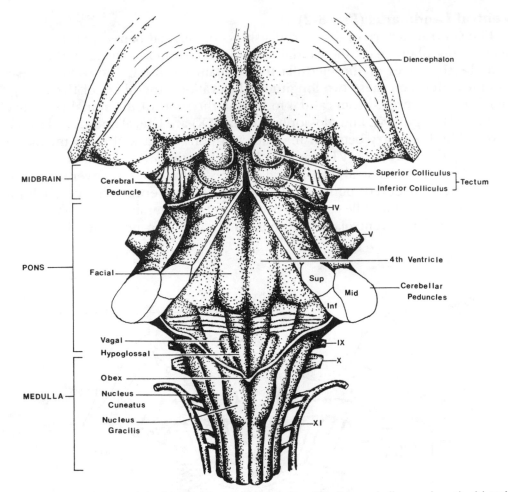

Figure 8-1. Dorsal view of the brainstem and diencephalon with the cerebellum and cerebral hemispheres removed and the roof of the fourth ventricle open. Cranial nerves are numbered.

the medulla. The vagal trigones (dorsal motor nucleus of cranial nerve X) lie just laterally and slightly caudally to the hypoglossal trigones. Almost the entire dorsal surface of the pons is covered by either the floor of the fourth ventricle or the cerebellar peduncles. Rostrally, the center of the pons is covered by the superior velum of the fourth ventricle. The paired facial colliculi can be seen in the floor of the fourth ventricle at the caudal end of the pons, just rostral to the hypoglossal trigones. The transversely cut inferior, middle, and superior cerebellar peduncles outline the fourth ventricle. The trochlear nerve (IV) marks the boundary between the pons and the midbrain. The dorsal surface of the midbrain is distinguished clearly by the paired inferior and superior colliculi constituting the corpora quadrigemina. The dorsal surfaces of the cerebral peduncles form the lateral boundary of the midbrain.

Ventral Landmarks (Fig. 8-2)

The ventral surface of the medulla shows the medial paired pyramids; the decussating fibers mark the caudal limit of the medulla. Lateral to the pyramids lie the olives of the medulla that contain the inferior olivary nuclear complex. Between these two longitudinal elevations, the fibers of the hypoglossal nerve emerge. From caudal to rostral, the roots of the spinal accessory nerve (XI), vagus (X), and glossopharyngeal (IX) are lateral and dorsal to the olives. The boundary between medulla and pons is marked from medial to lateral by the abducens (VI), facial (VII), and vestibulocochlear (VIII) nerve roots. The entire ventral and lateral surface of the pons is covered by the transversely oriented pontocerebellar fibers that enter the cerebellum through the large middle cerebral peduncle. The trigeminal nerve (V) penetrates these fibers ventrolaterally about midway in the pons. At the caudal

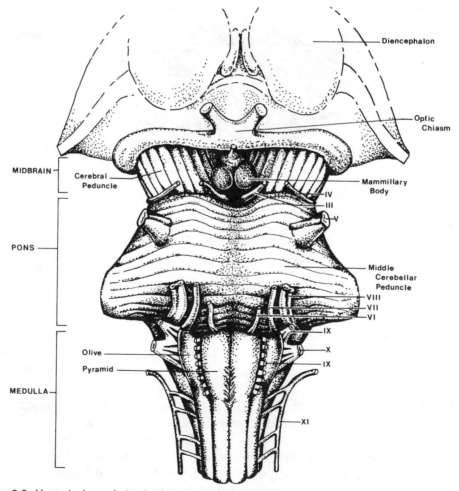

Figure 8-2. Ventral view of the brainstem and diencephalon with the cerebral hemispheres and cerebellum removed. Cranial nerves are numbered.

extent of the midbrain, the fibers of the oculomotor nerve (III) emerge near the midline. The remainder of the ventral midbrain is distinguished by the longitudinal fibers of the basis pedunculi (cerebral peduncles) that contain the corticospinal, corticobulbar, and corticopontine tracts. The rostral extent of the midbrain is not defined clearly either ventrally or dorsally because of the complex folding of structures) related to the presence of the cephalic flexure and the enlargement of the diencephalon.

General Organization of the Brainstem Grey Matter

The nuclear columns mentioned earlier bear a constant relationship to each other throughout the extent of the brain stem, even though some of them are discontinuous. The basic arrangement is illustrated in Figure 8-3. It is impor-

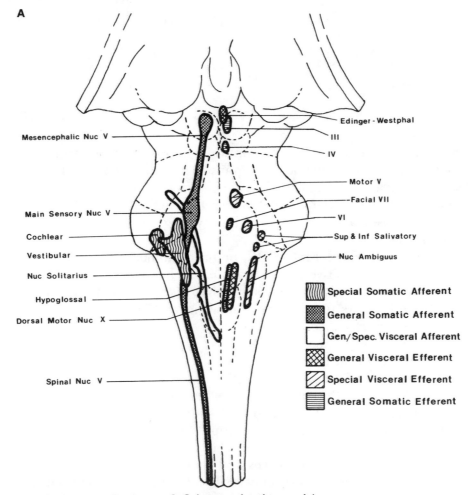

Figure 8-3. Brainstem cell columns. **A.** Columns related to cranial nerves.

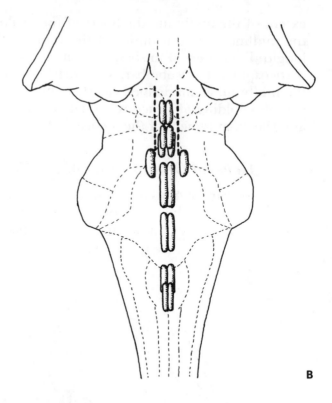

Figure 8-3.
B. Raphe nuclei. The dotted region in the midbrain represents the periaqueductal grey region of the midbrain reticular formation.

tant to note that the sulcus limitans continues to provide a consistent demarcation between sensory and motor regions. The motor nuclei of the cranial nerves in the brainstem are classified as follows:

1. General somatic motor (GSE) innervating somatic skeletal muscle.
2. General visceral efferent (GVE) innervating smooth muscle, glands and the heart.
3. Special visceral efferent (SVE), or branchiomeric, innervating striated skeletal muscle derived from branchial arches.

The motor nuclei are organized somewhat discretely; that is, one nucleus generally sends fibers to only one cranial nerve. The sensory nuclei of the cranial nerves are classified as follows:

1. General somatic afferent (GSA).
2. Special somatic afferent (SSA).
3. General visceral afferent (GVA).
4. Special visceral afferent (SVA).

Sensory nuclei are organized functionally rather than anatomically; that is, a given nucleus or part of a nucleus will represent one sense modality and may collect relevant information from a number or cranial nerves. The motor and sensory nuclei of the cranial nerves and their functions are summarized in Table 8-3. Special sensory cranial nerves I and II have been omitted from this discussion because their primary afferents do not enter the brainstem. Effer-

TABLE 8-3. Classification of Cranial Nerves and Brainstem Nuclei by Functional Fiber Type

Fiber Type	Structures Innervated	Nuclei	Cranial Nerves
GSE	muscles derived from myotomes	oculomotor trochlear abducens hypoglossal	III IV VI XII
SVE	muscles derived from branchial arches	motor nuc. of V facial nuc. ambiguus spinal nuc. of XI	V VII IX,X,(XI) XI
GVE	smooth muscle, glands, myocardium	Edinger-Westphal nuc. sup. salivatory nuc. inf. salivatory nuc. dorsal motor nuc. of X	III VII IX X
GSA	skin of face and mucous membranes of mouth: · pain and temperature · discriminatory touch muscles of face, jaw and eye: · proprioception	 spinal nuc. of V main sensory nuc. of V mesencephalic nuc. of V	 V, IX, X V,VII,IX,X V,VII(?),III(?)
SSA	sensory organs of inner ear: · vestibular sensation · auditory sensation	 vestibular nuclei cochlear nuclei	 VIII (vest.) VIII (cochlear)
GVA	internal organs: · pain, pressure, chemoreception	 nucleus solitarius	 IX, X
SVA	taste buds: · taste	 nucleus solitarius	 VII, IX, X
Receptor Regulatory	auditory hair cells m. stapedius m. tensor tympani vestibular hair cells muscle spindles	superior olive facial motor n. V ? all GSE and SVE nuclei	VIII VII V VIII all GSE and SVE nerves

ent fibers providing regulation of the behaviors of sensory receptors are located in cranial nerve VIII (both components) and in the general and special somatic efferent nerves (gamma motor neurons to muscle spindles).

Contents of Brainstem Regions

Medulla (Fig. 8-4)

The most caudal region of the brainstem, the medulla, contains sensory and motor nuclei related to the 9th through 12th cranial nerves (glossopharyngeal, vagus, hypoglossal, and spinal accessory) and a major portion of the spinal sensory nucleus of the 5th (trigeminal) nerve. The inferior vestibular nucleus is contained partly in the rostral portion of the medulla. Additionally, the medulla contains a major motor-system integration nucleus, the inferior olivary nuclear complex. Dorsally in the caudal medulla there are two sensory relay nuclei: the nucleus gracilis and the nucleus cuneatus. Ascending dorsal

Figure 8-4. Major components of the medulla (shown unilaterally). *CST,* corticospinal tract, *DSC,* dorsal spinocerebellar tract, *ML,* medial lemniscus, *MLF,* medial longitudinal fasciculus, *NA,* nucleus ambiguus, *SN,* solitary nucleus, *ST (on right side),* solitary tract, *ST (on left side),* spinothalamic tracts, *TS,* tectospinal tract, *TT,* trigeminothalamic tract, *VSC,* ventral spinocerebellar tract, *V(S),* spinal nucleus and tract of the trigeminal nerve, *VIII,* vestibular nuclear area, *X,* dorsal motor nucleus of the vagus, *XII,* hypoglossal nucleus. The inferior olivary nuclear complex which occupies the ventral half of the medulla has been omitted for clarity.

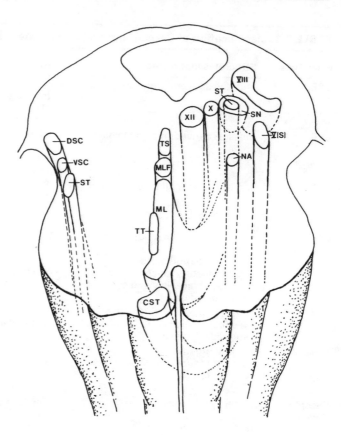

column fibers synapse in these nuclei. Projecting fibers from the nuclei run ventrally and decussate (decussation of the medial lemniscus) to form the ascending medial lemniscus. Other ascending spinal tracts, particularly the spinocerebellar, spinothalamic, and spinotectal tracts, are positioned laterally the length of the medulla. The posterior spinocerebellar tract exits the medulla at its rostral extent to enter the inferior cerebellar peduncle. The pyramids located ventrally and medially contain the descending corticospinal fibers that decussate near the caudal end of the medulla and come to lie laterally in the cervical spinal cord. The tectospinal tract and the medial longitudinal fasciculus containing the medial vestibulospinal tract are located in the midline dorsal to the medial lemniscus. Other descending tracts are located laterally and somewhat ventrally, generally central to any ascending tract fibers.

Pons (Fig. 8-5)

The pons is divided into a dorsally placed tegmentum and a ventrally placed base. The base of the pons contains relatively few components: numerous scattered pontine nuclei that have a motor system relay function, fibers projecting from these nuclei into the middle cerebellar peduncles, and the dispersed descending corticospinal and corticobulbar fibers to medullary cranial nerves. Corticopontine fibers that have descended to the pons in

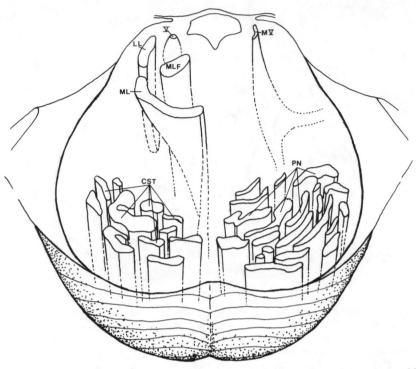

Figure 8-5. Major components of the pons (shown unilaterally). *LL,* lateral lemniscus, *ML,* medial lemniscus, *MLF,* medial longitudinal fasciculus, *MV,* motor nucleus of the trigeminal nerve, *PN,* pontine nuclei, *V,* principle sensory nucleus of the trigeminal nerve corticospinal tract.

company with the corticospinal and corticobulbar fibers terminate in the pontine nuclei. The tegmentum of the pons contains motor and sensory nuclei for the 5th through 8th (trigeminal, abducens, facial, and vestibulocochlear) cranial nerves. Additional sensory relay nuclei related to the auditory system also are located in the pontine tegmentum. The major ascending tracts, medial lemniscus, spinothalamic, and lateral lemniscus (an auditory system tract) are located in a band between the tegmentum and the base of the pons from medial to lateral. A major brainstem tract, the central tegmental tract, is located centrally in the tegmentum.

Midbrain (Fig. 8-6)

The midbrain is also divided into major segments: a base, a tegmental area, and the tectum. The base contains predominantly the corticospinal, corticobulbar, and corticopontine tracts collected in the cerebral peduncles, or basis pedunculi. Just dorsal to the peduncles lies the substantia nigra, a component of the basal ganglia, with predominantly motor relay function. Above the substantia nigra is the tegmentum that contains nuclei for the 3rd and 4th (oculomotor and trochlear) cranial nerves and the remaining ascending and descending tracts. The tegmentum contains the red nucleus, the final major motor relay nucleus of the brainstem. The tectum of the midbrain contains

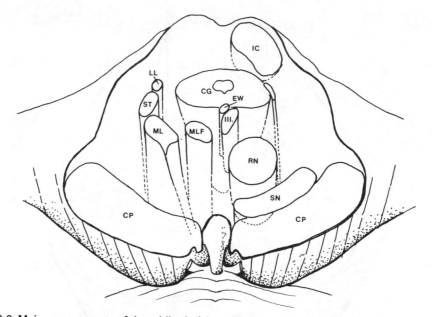

Figure 8-6. Major components of the midbrain (shown unilaterally). *CG,* central (periaqueductal) grey, *CP,* cerebral peduncles, *EW,* Edinger-Westphal nucleus, *IC,* inferior colliculus, *LL,* lateral lemniscus, *ML,* medial lemniscus, *MLF,* medial longitudinal fasciculus, *RN,* red nucleus, *SN,* substantia nigra, *ST,* spinothalamic tract, *III,* oculomotor nucleus.

the inferior and superior colliculi. The inferior colliculi are relay nuclei for the auditory system; the superior colliculi are relay nuclei for the visual motor system. Surrounding the Aqueduct of Sylvius is the central gray matter (periaqueductal gray) of the midbrain, which is a specialized part of the brainstem reticular formation.

Brainstem Reticular Formation

The remainder of the cellular material of the brainstem is located in the reticular formation, a widespread network of more or less extensively interconnected cells. Despite the apparent diffuse arrangement of cells in this system, there evidently is a very definite functional cellular organization that probably is associated with biochemical differentiation in terms of neurotransmitters.

Reticular neuron cell bodies are found in the midline and spread laterally and ventrally throughout the medulla and the tegmentum of the pons and midbrain. Generally, reticular cells can be clustered in three groups: 1) relatively well-defined midline (raphe) nuclei (Fig. 8-7), 2) an immediately adjacent large-celled region, and 3) a more laterally and ventrally placed small-celled region. These anatomical divisions do not always correspond very closely with functional divisions.

There are five major functions that can be identified with the reticular system:

1. Control of states of consciousness.
2. Modulation of learning.
3. Modulation of alpha and gamma motor neuron excitability.
4. Regulation of certain automatic, homeostatic functions such as heart rate and contractility, blood pressure, breathing rate and breathing volume.
5. Modulation of pain sensation.

The relationship between these functions and the anatomical and biochemical identification of the cells involved is indicated generally in Table 8-4. The reticular formation in the medulla is involved primarily with cardiovascular and respiratory function regulation and control of the general state of excitability of skeletal muscle alpha and gamma motor neurons. The pontine reticular formation also is involved in respiratory function regulation and probably to a certain extent in skeletal muscle neuron regulation. Cells in the upper pons are involved in controlling states of consciousness and in modulation of learning (locus coeruleus). The reticular formation of the midbrain has particularly been identified with control of states of consciousness and regulation of pain sensation.

The reticular formation is connected to the spinal cord through ascending spinoreticular tracts and various descending reticulospinal tracts. The portions of the reticular formation which are involved in regulation of cardiovascular and respiratory system activity are connected with the hypothalamus through various pathways including the central tegmental tract and the dorsal longitudinal fasciculus. There appears to be a definite potential for interconnections among functional systems within the reticular formation, as has been well demonstrated, particularly for the cardiovascular and respiratory systems.

TABLE 8-4. Functional Divisions of the Brainstem Reticular Formation

Function	Location of Cells in Reticular Formation	Putative Neurotransmitter(s)
Arousal	midbrain and upper pons	epinephrine or norepinephrine
Sleep	raphe nuclei, particularly in caudal pons nucleus of solitary tract	serotonin serotonin
Learning	locus coeruleus	norepinephrine
Motor Neuron Modulation	gigantocellular nucleus of medulla caudal pontine reticular nuclei	glutamate (?) glutamate (?)
Cardiovascular System Regulation	medullary reticular formation	epinephrine or norepinephrine
Respiratory System Regulation	medullary and caudal pontine reticular formation	epinephrine or norepinephrine
Pain Modulation in: Dorsal Horn Thalamus	raphe nuclei and periaqueductal grey periaqueductal grey	serotonin, enkephalins, substance P enkephalins (?)

Review Exercises

8-1.   Localize the following sensory modalities to the region of the brainstem (midbrain, pons or medulla) and the cranial nerve nucleus to which their primary afferent fibers project:

- auditory sensation
- vestibular sensation
- taste
- muscle stiffness in jaw muscles
- pain in the region of the eye

8-2.   As will be discussed in Chapter 9, vestibular sensory information is used to reflexively adjust the position of the eyes through activation of extrinsic eye muscles. Which nuclei in the brainstem are essential for this type of reflex activity to occur normally? Which brainstem tract(s) is (are) most likely to be involved in communicating the necessary information?

8-3.   Structural Models

Three dimensional models, including major landmarks, can be constructed for the following:

- a. dorsal column-medial lemniscus system showing nuclei and decussation
- b. pyramidal tract
- c. cranial nerves with autonomic motor function (GVE nuclei)
- d. cranial nerves with somatic and branchiomeric motor function (GSE and SVE nuclei)

9

Brainstem Sensory Systems: Trigemal, Gustatory, Cochlear, and Vestibular

The brainstem receives sensory information that is in many ways analogous to that received by the spinal cord. The trigeminal (5th cranial) nerve system provides skin and proprioceptive information from the face and jaws. The vestibular (8th cranial) nerve provides special kinesthetic information about the location and movement of the head in relationship to accelerating forces, typically gravity. The auditory (8th cranial) nerve provides hearing sensation, and fibers in the facial (7th cranial), glossopharyngeal (9th cranial), and vagus (Xth cranial) nerves provide special chemoreceptor information from the taste buds of the oral cavity. Visceral sensory information carried by the glossopharyngeal and vagus nerves will be discussed with other aspects of homeostatic regulation in Chapter 16.

Trigeminal Sensory System

The trigeminal nerve is the predominant somesthetic cranial nerve. Its functional and anatomical subdivisions, outlined in Table 9-1, include a principal sensory nucleus for epicritic (discrete) touch modalities, a spinal nucleus for protopathic modalities, a mesencephalic nucleus for proprioception and a small motor nucleus (Fig. 9-1).

The principal sensory nucleus of cranial nerve V correlates functionally with the nuclei gracilis and cuneatus of the dorsal column system. Both systems carry epicritic touch and proprioceptive information. Most secondary fibers from the principal sensory nucleus decussate within the pons at the level

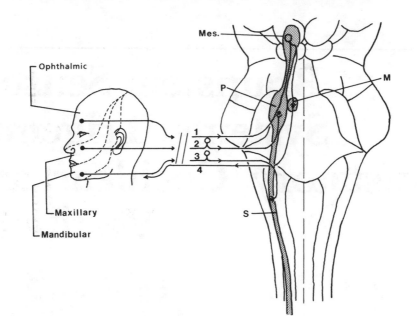

Figure 9-1. Trigeminal nerve (cranial nerve V). There are three peripheral divisions innervating the face, the ophthalmic, the maxillary and the mandibular. The mandibular division carries efferent somatosensory fibers *(4)* to jaw muscles. Three major types of sensory information are delivered from each of the peripheral divisions: proprioception *(1)* epicritic sensation *(2)* and protopathic sensation *(3)*. Fibers for epicritic and protopathic sensation have their cell bodies in the semilunar ganglion. Proprioceptive fiber cell bodies are located in the mesencephalic nucleus of V *(Mes.)*. Epicritic sensation is projected predominantly to the principal sensory nucleus of V *(P)* located in the mid pons. Protopathic sensation is projected to the spinal nucleus of V *(S)* which is continuous from the pons to the upper cervical spinal cord. The motor fibers have their cell bodies in the motor nucleus *(M)* which is adjacent to the principal sensory nucleus.

of the nucleus and project adjacent to the medial lemniscus through the ventral trigeminal tract. A separate, more medially located bundle, the dorsal trigeminal tract, carries uncrossed fibers. Both projections terminate within the ventral posterior (medial) nucleus of the thalamus. The information transmitted in the primary trigeminal system is projected from the thalamus to terminate somatotopically near the Sylvian fissure.

The spinal nucleus and tract of the trigeminal nerve correlate closely in function with the spinothalamic system, although the most cranial region of the spinal nucleus also receives discrete sensory information. Otherwise, the sensory modalities are the same, and the location of fibers and synapses is analogous to that described for the spinothalamic tracts. After entering the CNS and before synapsing, the primary afferent fibers course in Lissauer's tract of the cord or the tract of the spinal nucleus of V. The first synapse is in either the spinal nucleus of V or laminae II and III of the cervical spinal cord. The spinal nucleus of V is organized somatotopically, with afferents from the uppermost (opthalmic) division of the trigeminal nerve terminating in the upper levels of the nucleus, and afferents from the lowest (mandibular)

TABLE 9-1. Basic Functional Divisions of the Trigeminal Nuclei

Nucleus	Function	Afferent Connections	Efferent Connections
Principal Sensory	pressure, vibration, discriminatory touch sensation	1° afferents from all branches of V	2° uncrossed and crossed fibers through dorsal trigeminal tract and ventral trigeminal lemniscus to VPM of thalamus
Spinal	light touch, pain, temperature sensation	1° afferents from all branches of V by way of spinal tract of V	2° mainly crossed fibers through ventral trigeminal tract to VPM of thalamus
Mesencephalic	proprioception	1° afferent peripheral precesses by way of mesencephalic tract of V	· 1° afferent central processes to motor nucleus V by way of mesencephalic tract of V · 1° afferent central processes to cerebellum by way of sup. cer. ped.
Motor	activation of muscles of mastication	· 1° afferent central processes from mesencephalic nucleus of V (monosynaptic) · corticobulbar fibers and other motor control fibers	III (mandibular) branch of V

division terminating within the cervical cord. Projections of the spinal nucleus of V to the thalamus are predominantly crossed and lie closely adjacent to the projection of the spinothalamic tract (ventral trigeminal tract); both systems also send branches into the brainstem reticular formation (Fig. 9-2). The termination point in the thalamus is in the ventral posterior nucleus for both systems; body sensation is projected laterally and face sensation is projected medially.

The mesencephalic nucleus of the trigeminal nerve correlates functionally with Clarke's nucleus in the spinal cord (Fig. 9-3). Both project proprioceptive information to the cerebellum: Clarke's nucleus by way of the dorsal spinocerebellar tract and the mesencephalic nucleus by way of the superior cerebellar peduncle. The main difference between these two systems lies in the number of synapses involved. In the mesencephalic system, the first synapse is in the cerebellum instead of in the nucleus. Cells in the mesencephalic nucleus correspond to proprioceptive primary afferent cells found in spinal dorsal root ganglia. Myotatic reflexes (eg, jaw jerk) mediated by this system use monosynaptic connections between primary Ia afferents having their cell bodies in the mesencephalic nucleus and alpha motor neurons with cell bodies located in the motor nucleus of the trigeminal nerve.

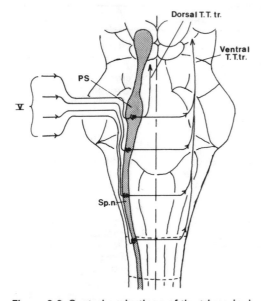

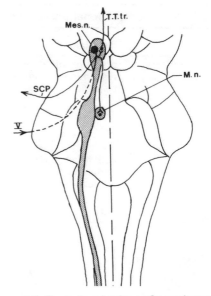

Figure 9-2. Central projections of the trigeminal system. Epicritic modalities (discriminatory touch) entering the principal sensory nucleus *(PS)* project bilaterally in the dorsal trigeminothalamic tract *(Dorsal T.T. tr.)* and the ventral trigeminothalamic tract *(Ventral T.T. tr.)*. Protopathic modalities (pain, temperature, general touch) entering the spinal nucleus *(Sp.n.)* project primarily contralateral but to a certain extent ipsilaterally, in the same tracts.

Figure 9-3. Central projections of proprioceptive information carried over the trigeminal nerve. The primary afferent cell bodies are in the mesencephalic nucleus *(Mes.n.)*. The central limb of these neurons projects to the motor nucleus *(M.n.)*. Additional projections from the mesencephalic nucleus are directed to the cerebellum over the superior cerebellar peduncle *(SCP)* and to the thalamus over the trigeminothalamic tracts *(T.T.tr.)*.

Gustatory System

Taste sensation is carried into the brainstem over the facial nerve (anterior two-thirds of the tongue), glossopharyngeal nerve (posterior one-third of the tongue), and vagus nerve (pharynx) (Fig. 9-4). Cell bodies of taste primary afferent fibers are located in the geniculate ganglion of the facial nerve, the petrosal ganglion of the glossopharyngeal nerve, and the nodose ganglion of the vagus nerve. The central termination of these primary afferents is predominantly in the upper portion of the nucleus of the solitary tract or the adjacent medullary reticular formation. Autonomic reflexes, such as salivation, elicited by taste sensation are organized within the reticular formation. The motor limb of the reflex begins in the superior and inferior salivatory nuclei, with peripheral projections in the facial and glossopharyngeal nerves (parasympathetic) and the upper thoracic spinal nerves (sympathetic). Central projections from the solitary nucleus carry taste information to the cerebral hemispheres by way of the ventral posterior medial nucleus of the thalamus. Additional projections subserving automatic responses to taste terminate in the hypothalamus and portions of the limbic system.

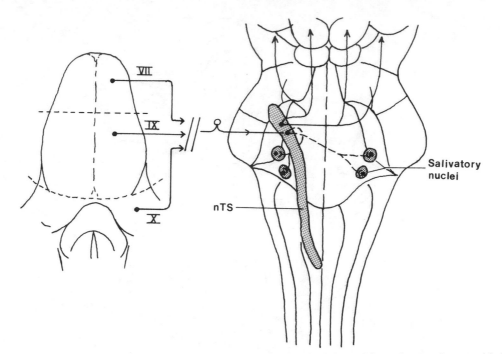

Figure 9-4. Pathways for gustatory sensation. Taste sensation is delivered from the anterior one-third of the tongue by the facial nerve (VII), from the posterior two-thirds of the tongue by the glossopharyngeal nerve (IX) and from the pharynx by the vagus nerve (X). All taste sensation is projected to the cranial portion of the nucleus of the solitary tract (nTS) in the pons. From this location reflex pathways regulating salivation project to the superior and inferior salivatory nuclei. Cranially-projecting pathways close to the trigeminothalamic tracts carry taste information bilaterally to the thalamus (VPM nucleus). From that location projections to the cortex provide a substrate for taste perception.

Auditory System

The auditory system exemplifies a number of the receptor and central coding characteristics described earlier as being the basis for precise sensory discrimination. The receptor itself is mechanically complex and designed to permit discrimination of both tone intensity and frequency (pitch) (Fig. 9-5). Receptor hair cells are embedded in the basilar membrane of the cochlea. This membrane vibrates in response to pressure waves delivered at the oval window. Frequency response of the membrane decreases regularly from the end closest to the window to the end at the tip of the cochlea. The hair cells thus are positioned in such a way as to produce initial tonotopic coding of auditory stimuli. In addition, the hair cells themselves are differentially sensitive to different rates of vibration. The tonotopic coding thus becomes transmitted by means of location coding by labeled lines. Within the cochlear nucleus where the central processes of the cells of the spiral (cochlear) ganglion terminate, location coding persists (Fig. 9-6). Ipsilateral projections and terminations of auditory information to the temporal lobe of the cerebral hemisphere are also tonotopically coded. Auditory sensory information is

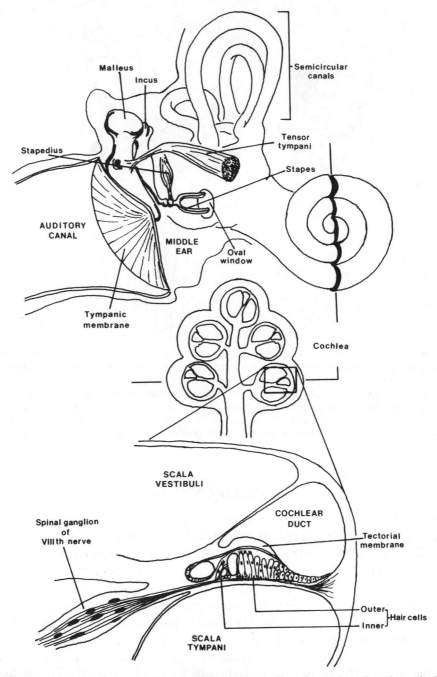

Figure 9-5. Components of the peripheral auditory system. *Top.* Coronal section through the skull showing structures of the middle and inner ear. The middle ear muscles, the stapedius and the tensor tympani, attach to the walls of the middle ear. The cochlea of the inner ear projects anterior to the plane of section. *Middle.* Section through the spiral cochlea showing the arrangement of the inner ear spaces and membranes. *Bottom.* Detailed section of the sensory apparatus of the cochlea. The spiral ganglion is contained within the central hollow bony core of the cochlea.

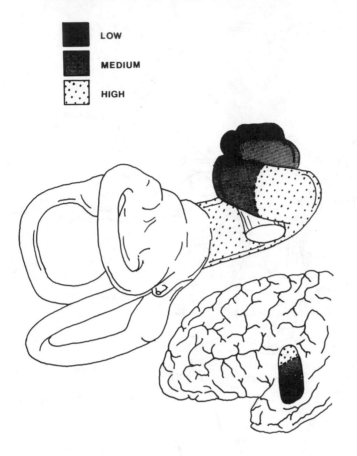

■ LOW

▨ MEDIUM

▨ HIGH

Figure 9-6. Tonotopic coding of the auditory system. Low frequency sounds are detected in the most flexible upper region of the cochlea while higher frequency sounds are detected in stiffer regions closer to the oval window. This relative spatial organization of frequency is maintained in the central auditory projections up to the level of cortical regions 41 and 42.

projected both ipsilaterally and contralaterally within the brainstem, with several synapses before projection from the thalamus to the cerebral hemispheres (Fig. 9-7). The ipsilateral projections appear to be the primary pathway for pitch and tone quality information. One apparent purpose of the crossed projections is discrimination of sound direction and movement through comparison of information received in both ears. Differences in auditory perceptual ability of the left and right cerebral cortices may be dependent on either subcortical decussations or cortical commissures, or both.

Like muscle spindles, the auditory receptor mechanism can have its function modified through efferent control pathways (Fig. 9-8). Efferent fibers originating in the superior olivary nucleus and carried in the 8th nerve serve to modulate the receptor sensitivity of the cochlear hair cells, thus permitting selective reception of specific tones. Efferent fibers carried in the facial nerve innervate the stapedius muscle while fibers in the trigeminal nerve innervate the tensor tympani. Contraction of the tensor tympani muscle stiffens the tympanic membrane, causing increased sensitivity to high frequency sound waves. The control of hair cell and tympanic membrane function serves primarily sensory discriminatory function and as such has complex cortical regulation. Contraction of the stapedius muscle stiffens the chain of middle

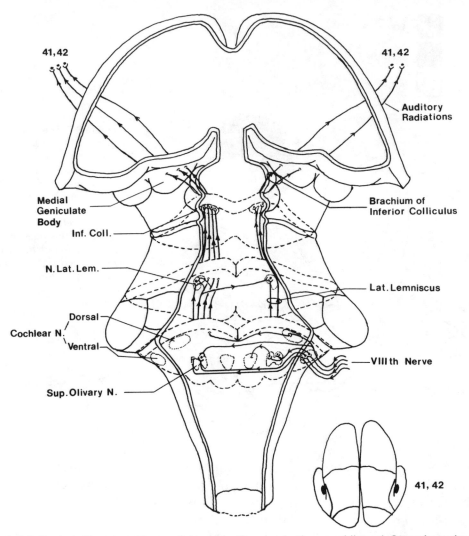

Figure 9-7. Central afferent auditory pathways. Auditory projections are bilateral. Commissural transmission occurs in the brainstem predominantly at the level of entry in the pons and slightly higher at the level of the nucleus of the lateral lemniscus *(N. Lat. Lem.)*. Commissural projections (not shown) also connect the two inferior colliculi *(Inf. Coll.)*. Processed auditory information is transmitted between the two hemispheres via the corpus collosum.

ear ossicles and lessens the impact of the stapes on the round window, thus decreasing the volume of the vibrations generated in the cochlea. The stapedius reflex elicited by high noise volume is probably a monosynaptic reflex with the substrate entirely contained in the lower pons. It is a unilateral reflex, but it can spread to both ears with sufficiently high sound intensity. The reflex is used clinically to give a general assessment of both 8th and 7th nerve function. This efferent control of the auditory sensory system is activated also during normal speech.

The auditory brainstem projection pathways are also the basis for addition-

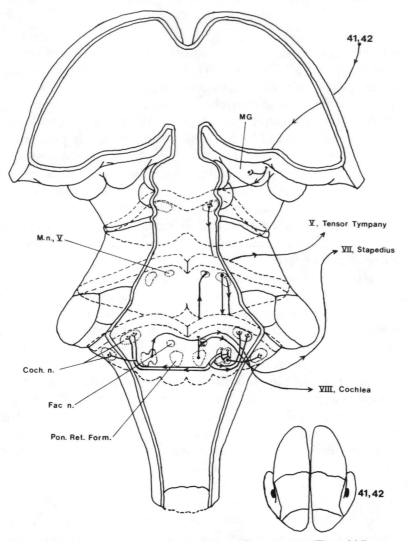

Figure 9-8. Efferent sensory control projections of the auditory system. The middle ear muscles are controlled by the trigeminal nerve (V) projecting to the tensor tympani and the facial nerve (VII) projecting to the stapedius. Sensitivity of cochlear hair cells is regulated by projections in the cochlear portion of the eighth nerve. The superior olivary nucleus is a major coordinating center for auditory efferent control. Corticobulbar projections originating in areas 41 and 42 of the temporal lobe permit coordination of auditory sensitivity with conscious requirements for hearing. Control can be expressed bilaterally or unilaterally. *Coch. n.*, cochlear nuclei; *Fac. n.*, facial nucleus; *MG*, medial geniculate body; *M.n., V*, motor nucleus of V; *Pon. Ret. Form.*, pontine reticular formation.

al clinical tests used to evaluate the general status of the brainstem. Evoked auditory responses can be elicited through the presentation of specific tones and recorded superficially from skull electrodes. The pattern of evoked responses can be analyzed to evaluate the transmission of auditory information at each stage in the brainstem pathways. This information in turn can be used to give an estimate of the structural and functional integrity of surrounding brainstem structures.

Vestibular System

The vestibular receptors are located in the petrous portion of the temporal bone adjacent to the middle ear cavity (Fig. 9-9). The receptors are located in three mutually perpendicular canals and in an adjoining open area, the vestibule. In the normal head upright position, the anterior (superior) and posterior canals are in the vertical plane at 45° to the sagittal plane and perpendicular to each other. The horizontal canal is nearly perpendicular to the other two; it is angled upward 15° anteriorly. Anterior and posterior canals of opposite sides are in nearly parallel planes. The bony canals and vestibule are continuous with the cochlea of the inner ear. Within the bony structures lie the membranous canals surrounded by perilymph. The interior of the canals, vestibule, and cochlea is filled with endolymph. The endolymph spaces are continuous with each other and drain into the subarachnoid space through the endolymphatic duct.

The vestibular receptors are made up of hair cells with their cilia inserted into overlying gelatinous material. Within the canals, the hair cells are located in enlargements, called ampullae, that are nearly filled by the gelatinous cupola, allowing minimal passage of endolymph. The base of each ampulla is elevated into a crista (Fig. 9-10). The ampullae of the horizontal and anterior canals are located anteriorly, while that of the posterior canal is located posteriorly. The utricle of the vestibule lies in the horizontal plane; the saccule is in the vertical plane. The overlying gelatinous material for these receptors has small calcium carbonate crystals, or statoliths, embedded in it (Fig. 9-11). These statoliths have sufficient mass to cause displacement of the gelatinous material in response to gravity or any other constant accelerating force. The cilia of the hair cells have a directional orientation that permits generation of direction-specific response in the cells.

The vestibular nerve innervates the three ampullae and the utricle and saccule of the vestibule. Cell bodies for these primary afferent fibers are located in Scarpa's ganglion, which lies within the internal auditory meatus (Fig. 9-12). The vestibular nerve also contains regulatory efferent fibers that act to adjust the sensitivity of the hair cells to mechanical stimulation.

Upon entering the brainstem, the central processes of the vestibular nerve fibers are distributed to the vestibular nuclei and the cerebellum. The vestibular nuclei are located dorsolaterally in the brainstem at the level of the junction between the medulla and the pons. They include a superior, lateral, inferior, and medial collection of cells, each with distinct afferent and efferent connections. Fibers from the canals project to the superior nucleus and the anterior portion of the medial and inferior nuclei. Fibers from the utricle project to the adjacent portions of the medial and inferior nuclei; fibers from the saccula project to the lateral portion of the inferior nucleus. All fibers send projections to the lateral, or Deiter's, nucleus (Fig. 9-13).

The vestibular nuclei have extensive central connections that can be classed into three groups: descending projections to the spinal cord, ascending pro-

A

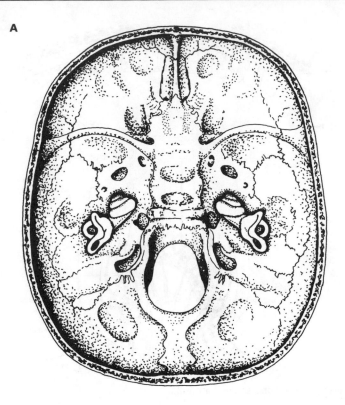

B

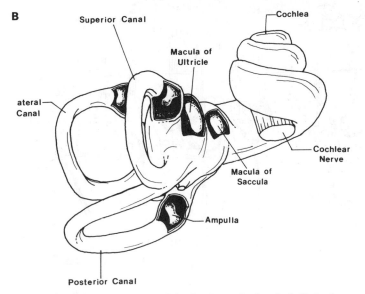

Superior Canal

Cochlea

Macula of
Ultricle

ateral
Canal

Cochlear
Nerve

Macula of
Saccula

Ampulla

Posterior Canal

Figure 9-9. Vestibular apparatus. **A.** Location of the inner ear in the skull. Note the parallelism of the superior and posterior canals of the two sides. **B.** Detail showing the location of the ampullae and maculae within the vestibular apparatus.

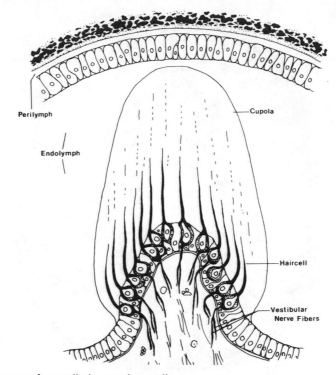

Figure 9-10. Cut-away of a vestibular canal ampulla.

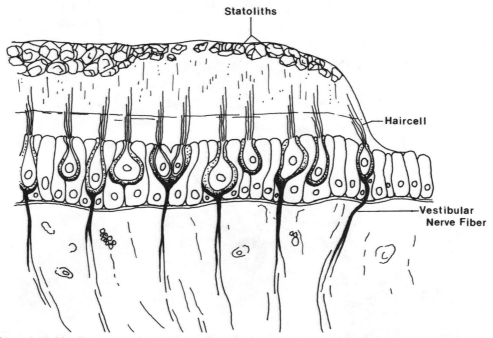

Figure 9-11. Vestibular macula. The haircell projections or cilia have a definite directional orientation which varies depending on the location of the cell within the macula. The longest, or kinocilium, is morphologically different from the other cilia.

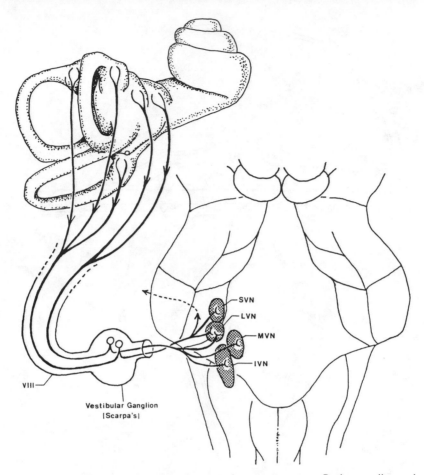

Figure 9-12. Vestibular nerve projections into the central nervous system. Both ampullar and macular receptors project their information to all vestibular nuclei in a definite and consistent pattern. This pattern is continued in projections from the vestibular nuclei to other central neural locations, in particular the cranial nerve nuclei related to extraocular muscles and the cervical spinal cord. Projections to the cerebellum over the inferior cerebellar peduncle may be primary afferent collaterals or secondary fibers arising in the vestibular nuclei. *IVN,* inferior vestibular nucleus, *LVN,* lateral (Deiter's) vestibular nucleus, *MVN,* medial vestibular nucleus, *SVN,* superior vestibular nucleus.

jections to the brainstem and thalamus, and cerebellar projections. Descending fibers arising from the lateral, or Deiter's, nucleus pass into the spinal cord through the lateral vestibulospinal tract, which extends the length of the spinal cord. Projections from the inferior and medial vestibular nuclei descend through the cervical levels of the cord in the medial longitudinal fasciculus. This pathway in the pons and midbrain carries the ascending projections from the medial and superior nuclei to the nuclei for the extraocular muscles, providing the substrate for vestibular-ocular reflex interaction. Vestibular nuclear projections to the vermis and flocculonodular lobe of the cerebellum pass through the inferior cerebellar peduncle. Many of the primary vestibular afferents also send direct branches to the cerebellum through

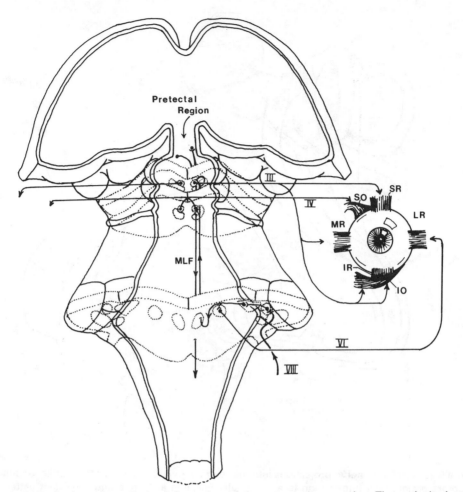

Figure 9-13. Projection of vestibular information to the extraocular muscles. The main brainstem transmission pathway permitting coordination of eye movement in response to vestibular information is the medial longitudinal fasciculus *(MLF)*. The abducens nerve (VI) controls the ipsilateral lateral rectus *(LR)*. The trochlear nerve (IV) controls the contralateral superior oblique *(SO)*. The remainder of the extraocular muscles, superior rectus *(SR)*, medial rectus *(MR)*, inferior oblique *(IO)*, and inferior rectus *(IR)* are controlled ipsilaterally by the oculomotor nerve (III). Vestibular information is projected bilaterally from the vestibular nuclei leading to coordinated control of both eyes (conjugate gaze).

this pathway. The vestibular nuclei of either side are connected reciprocally, permitting coordination of response to input from both vestibular organs. Normal operation of vestibular-directed motor behavior is dependent on congruent information from both organs. Discrepant information, such as can occur with peripheral vestibular pathology, or during some types of vestibular system testing (see below) can lead to abnormal perceptual and motor behavior such as nausea, vomiting, dizziness, and loss of coordination. Loss of input from one side, however, does not cause permanent disability.

Response Characteristics of Vestibular Receptors

The vestibular receptors are of two physiological types: rapidly adapting, or phasic, and slowly adapting, or tonic. The hair cells of the semicircular canals are rapidly adapting. When no stimulation is present they fire at a constant frequency. Bending of the hair cells as a result of relative movement between the endolymph and the walls of the canals elicits either hyperpolarization of the receptors with a concomitant decrease in firing frequency or relative depolarization with an increase in firing frequency. These receptors thus are an example of directionally specific receptors. Because of the physical properties of the canals and the endolymph, the hair cells are exposed to stimulation only during periods of acceleration and not during periods when the head is moving at a constant velocity. Signals from the ampullae inform the CNS either of initiation or cessation of head movement (in any plane) or of changes in the velocity of head movement; however, they do not provide information about constant head position or velocity.

The hair cells of the maculae are slowly adapting. They also have a constant resting firing frequency that is modified by stimulation. The effective stimulus for macular cells is deflection of the hairs in response to movement of the otolith membrane that results from gravitational or other accelerational forces. This stimulus is constant while the head is in any given position in relationship to the accelerating force. Because of their slowly adapting nature, macular cells can signal constant or tonic information concerning head position.

Vestibular Reflexes

The vestibular sensory system has strong reflex connections to 1) extraocular muscles, 2) neck muscles, 3) trunk muscles, and 4) proximal extremity muscles. The reflexes elicited by vestibular stimulation may be either phasic or tonic in nature, corresponding to the character of the sensory information. The reflexes involving neck and extraocular muscles serve primarily to maintain the head upright in respect to gravity and to stabilize the eyes during head movement. Reflexes involving trunk and proximal limb muscles position the trunk and proximal joints in relationship to the ground (gravity).

Vestibular-ocular reflex pathways are used to elicit conjugate gaze and nystagmus. Because the stimulus is head movement or position, visual input is not necessary and the responses occur with or without the eyes open. Conjugate gaze is a tonic reflex initiated by detected changes in head position and maintained by constant macular input. The eyes are moved together (in the same direction) in such a way as to maintain normal horizontal and vertical orientation of the visual fields on the retina. Conjugate gaze adjustments occur in all planes and include rotational movements of the eyes and lateral and vertical displacements.

Vestibular nystagmus is a phasic response to stimulation of ampullar hair cells. It occurs in response to accelerations of the head and is not seen when the head is at rest or moving with constant velocity. Nystagmus has a slow, initial eye movement component and a subsequent fast recovery component. The slow component consists of conjugate deviation of the eyes in the direction of endolymph movement and hair cell deflection (*opposite* to the direction of head movement). As the eyes reach the limit of movement in this initial direction, they are returned to midline (or past) by a fast saccadic movement in the direction of head movement. The direction of nystagmus is named by the direction of the saccade, probably because this movement is more evident to the observer. Vestibular nystagmus enables the eyes to maintain fixation on objects that are stationary in respect to the moving head. As is true during all saccadic movements, visual sensory information is not processed centrally during the saccades of vestibular nystagmus. Vestibular nystagmus can be elicited by any stimulus causing relative movement of the endolymph and the walls of the canals. Clinically, vestibular nystagmus can be induced either by rotating the subject or by differentially warming or cooling the endolymph through introduction of water into the outer ear. In rotational testing nystagmus is observed typically at the cessation of rotation (postrotatory nystagmus) when the head can be stabilized for observation. Caloric testing has the disadvantage of being an abnormal and unilateral stimulus. As such, it tends to cause responses associated with any stimuli that provide conflicting vestibular and ocular information to the brainstem. Electrical stimulation of the vestibular nerve also can induce nystagmus.

Nystagmus may also be observed with the eyes open when the head is stationary and the external world is moving in a uniform direction. This *optokinetic* nystagmus also serves to permit visual fixation of objects; it has the same components of conjugate deviation followed by a saccade. The conjugate deviation is in the direction of the moving object. In testing for nystagmus and other vestibular reflexes, the eyes of the subject must be closed while the stimulus is presented to avoid the introduction of visual reflexes.

Both conjugate gaze and vestibular nystagmus are mediated by connections between the vestibular nuclei and the extraocular muscle nuclei (abducens, trochlear, and oculomotor). The information is carried by the medial longitudinal fasciculus. The coordination of visual and vestibular information normally involved in producing visual fixation with recovery saccades occurs in an area of the pontine reticular formation immediately adjacent to the abducens nucleus. There is a strict direction-specific projection from pairs of vestibular canals to pairs of extraocular muscles controlling eye movement in each eye (Fig. 9-13).

Labyrinthine Reflexes Acting on the Neck and Body

Vestibular (labyrinthine) information concerning head position or movement relative to gravity is used in both phasic and tonic reflexes to orient the head and body relative to gravity. The phasic, or labyrinthine righting reflexes, act predominantly on neck muscles. They serve to maintain the face vertical in the presence of head displacements out of the upright position (Fig. 9-14). Head acceleration stimuli act on the ampullae of the appropriate canals that then send the information to the vestibular nuclei. From here, appropriate activating signals are sent bilaterally to the neck muscle motor neurons through the descending portion of the medial longitudinal fasciculus. Al-

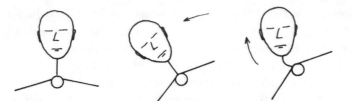

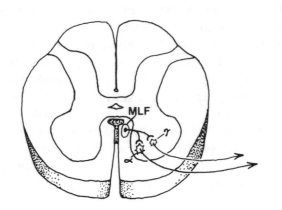

Figure 9-14. Labyrinthine righting reflex. Shown as a response to lateral flexion of the body, this reflex also acts with displacement in all other directions to return the head to the upright position. The effectors involved are the neck muscles which are controlled by way of projection of vestibular information through the descending portion of the medial longitudinal fasciculus *(MLF)*.

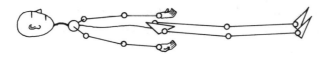

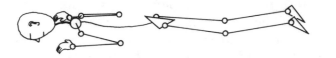

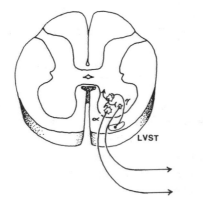

Figure 9-15. Tonic labyrinthine reflex. Sustained stimulation of the maculae produce extension of the trunk and extremities in the supine position (top) and flexion in the prone position (middle). These tonic postures can be marked when the descending vestibular information through the lateral vestibulospinal tract *(LVST)* is released from other CNS control. Both alpha and gamma motor neurons are controlled, probably through interneurons.

though the righting response is viewed typically as a phasic behavior, it has a static component initiated and maintained by macular input. This component serves to maintain the face vertical position once it has been attained.

Tonic labyrinthine responses to face (head) position relative to gravity can be observed in the muscles of the trunk and proximal extremities. The sensors for these responses are the maculae and the descending spinal pathway used is the lateral vestibulospinal tract (Fig. 9-15). In the face down position (neck flexion) this reflex system increases the level of excitation of alpha motor neurons to trunk and proximal extremity flexors. In the face up position (neck extension), extensor motor neuron excitation is increased. When the face is vertical (neck neutral), there is increased excitation of extensors of the trunk and lower extremities and of flexors of the upper extremities. Although we are not normally aware of the effect of tonic vestibular activation as adults, these shifts in alpha motor neuron excitation, like others embodied in primitive reflexes, are typically a part of the normal posture and movement repertoire. The reader can test for the presence of tonic labyrinthine reflexes by comparing the ease of maintaining an erect trunk posture in sitting or standing when the head is flexed forward, when it is upright, and when it is extended.

Review Exercises

9-1. Draw a wiring diagram for the "jaw jerk" reflex and compare it to that presented for the monosynaptic stretch reflex in Chapter 7. Include in your diagram additional central projections for the muscle spindle primary information.

9-2. Trigeminal neuralgia, sometimes termed "tic doloreux", results from pathology in the trigeminal nerve or semilunar ganglion. The symptoms are chronic, severe pain in one side of the face involving one or more of the branches of the trigeminal nerve. Identify locations at which pain sensation originating in the trigeminal nerve could be interrupted by surgical lesions. Consider adjacent structures and discuss which lesions would
   a. be most effective in permanently stopping the delivery of pain information to the thalamus.
   b. be least likely to affect the transmission of other sensory information from either the body or the face.

9-3. One common complaint of people using hearing aids to correct deafness is that they are no longer able to select which sounds to hear. Describe the normal mechanisms used by the auditory system which permit selective hearing and suggest why they are lacking in people with deafness and why hearing aids do not correct the problem. Consider the implications of this type of problem when treating patients with deafness.

9-4. Observation of vestibular reflexes. In all cases of observation, be sure that the subject (human) understands the tests and the responses which are likely to occur, and that the subject (human or animal) has indicated a willingness to participate. (Animals do have ways of indicating that they are not willing subjects.)

    a. Vestibular nystagmus. Position a human subject sitting on a rotating stool (available in most clinical laboratory settings). Have the subject close the eyes, and rotate the subject rapidly for 5-10 turns. Immediately upon ceasing rotation have the subject open the eyes while facing you. You should be able to observe horizontal nystagmus and identify the direction of the saccades. CAUTION: Do not prolong the rotation unnecessarily. In some subjects extended vestibular stimulation of this type can cause nausea.

    b. Vestibular righting reflexes can be observed easily in normally behaving infants at the age of 4-8 months and in cats. Remember, if the subject's eyes are open the vestibular and visual reflexes will both be operating and cannot be distinguished from each other.

        To observe vestibular righting reflexes, position the subject in the normal upright position (quadruped for cats) and tilt the head (or head and body together) in the sagittal and frontal planes.

    c. Tonic vestibular reflexes can be observed by positioning an infant or cat prone and supine. The easiest time to observe the reflexes is when the subject is asleep and has positioned itself naturally. The effect of tonic vestibular reflexes also may be observed in gymnasts and divers who use head movement and position to influence the posture of the body and proximal extremity joints.

9-5. Construct a diagram or model showing all of the components and connections involved in translating head rotation to the *left* into conjugate gaze to the *right*.

10

Basic Anatomy and Function of the Diencephalon

The diencephalon is immediately cranial to the midbrain, overlapping it both dorsally and laterally. The diencephalon, in turn, is surrounded completely by the enlarged cerebral hemispheres, except for a small ventral surface. In the midsagittal plane the diencephalon surrounds the laterally compressed third ventricle, forming its walls. The boundaries of the diencephalon are not clearly restricted to any one plane, and are formed of various tracts that connect the nuclear portions of the diencephalon with either the cerebral hemispheres or the brainstem (Fig. 10-1).

The diencephalon is subdivided into a number of major nuclear groups connected by a large number of fiber pathways. The major divisions of the diencephalon and their nuclei are as follows:

1. Epithalamus, containing the pineal body and habenular nuclei.
2. Dorsal thalamus (thalamus), containing numerous sensory and motor relay nuclei.
3. Hypothalamus, containing motor and integration nuclei dealing with homeostatic function.
4. Subthalamus, containing motor integration nuclei.

The epithalamus and hypothalamus, with their predominant homeostatic control functions, will be discussed in Chapter 15. The subthalamus will be discussed with the basal ganglia in Chapter 14. The thalamus proper, providing the major relay station between sensory systems and the cerebral hemispheres and being a relay point for motor integration pathways, will be discussed here.

Four major functions are carried out by the nuclei of the thalamus:

1. Integration and relay of sensory information from all afferent systems to the appropriate sensory receptor regions of the cerebral hemispheres.
2. Integration and relay of motor control information from the cerebellum and basal ganglia to the motor regions of the cerebral hemispheres.
3. Gating of passage of sensory and motor information.
4. Transmission of commands about the state of consciousness from the brainstem reticular formation to the cerebral hemispheres.

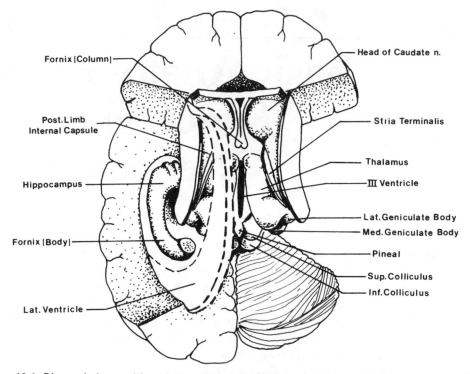

Figure 10-1. Diencephalon and its relationships viewed in horizontal section. The diencephalon sits within the curve formed by the lateral ventricle of each hemisphere. From this dorsal view only the thalamus and epithalamus (pineal) are visible. Fiber tracts which form boundaries for the diencephalon include the posterior limb of the internal capsule laterally, the stria terminalis dorsolaterally and the fornix dorsomedially.

Each nucleus within the thalamus has predominant relay functions and unique connections with the cortex and subcortical structures (Fig. 10-2). These functions can be listed as follows:

1. Relay of specific sensory or motor information (specific relay nuclei).
2. Relay of complex information that is neither purely motor nor purely sensory. The relay may be directed to specific, limited cortical regions (association nuclei), or diffusely projected to widespread cortical regions (diffuse nuclei).
3. Relay of information to noncortical components of the cerebral hemispheres (subcortical nuclei).

Many thalamic nuclei receive reciprocal innervation from their target areas. In addition to these functional divisions of the thalamus, the nuclei can be described in terms of their anatomical location. Groups of thalamic nuclei are separated from each other by fiber pathways. These anatomical groups include the following, from anterior to posterior within the thalamus:

1. Upper (dorsal) tier of nuclei: anterior, lateral dorsal, dorso medial, lateral posterior, pulvinar.

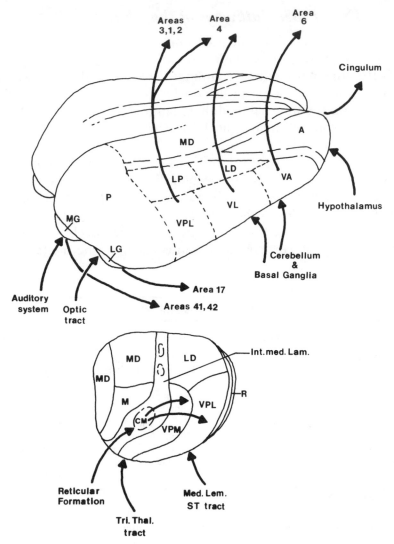

Figure 10-2. Major nuclei of the thalamus with their primary afferent and efferent relationships. *Top,* dorsolateral view of the paired thalamus. *Bottom,* cross-sectional view of one thalamus. The anterior nuclear group is enclosed within the branches of the intermedullary lamina. Internally this fiber bundle surrounds a number of functionally diffuse nuclei including the centromedian nucleus. *A,* anterior nuclear group; *CM,* centromedian n.; *LD,* lateral dorsal n.; *LP,* lateral posterior n.; *M,* medial nuclear group; *MD,* medial dorsal n.; *Md,* midline nuclei; *P,* pulvinar; *R,* reticular n.; *VA,* ventral anterior n.; *VL,* ventral lateral n.; *VPL,* ventral posterior lateral n.; *VPM,* ventral posterior medial n.

2. Lower (ventral) tier of nuclei: ventral anterior, ventral lateral, ventral posterior (lateral and medial regions).
3. Metathalamic nuclei (below and lateral to the pulvinar): geniculate bodies (lateral and medial).
4. Intralaminar (located within thalamus between tiers): centromedian.
5. Reticular nucleus located over most of lateral surface of the thalamus.

These major thalamic nuclei, their functional designation, and their location are summarized in Table 10-1.

Fiber Pathways of the Thalamus

Lying among various thalamic nuclei are thin fiber bundles that predominantly carry connecting fibers between various nuclei. The largest of these bundles is the internal medullary lamina. Posteriorly, this pathway separates the pulvinar and ventral posterior nuclei from the dorsomedial nucleus. Embedded within the internal medullary lamina is the centromedian nucleus. Anteriorly, this group of fibers splits to provide medial and lateral boundaries for the anterior nucleus.

The very large internal capsule with its caudal continuation, the cerebral peduncles, surrounds the thalamus laterally, anteriorly, dorsally and to a certain extent ventroposteriorly. The internal capsule contains fibers projecting from thalamic nuclei to the cerebral hemispheres (and their reciprocal fibers, when present) and fibers passing from the cerebral hemispheres to form the corticospinal, corticobulbar, and corticopontine tracts. Seen in hori-

TABLE 10-1 Function and Location of Major Thalamic Nuclei

Nucleus	Location	Afferents From	Projection To
Specific Relay Nuclei			
Anterior (A)	anterior	anterior hypothalamus	· cingulate gyrus · hippocampus
Ventral Lateral (VL)	ventral tier	· basal ganglia · cerebellum	· cortex area 4
Ventral Anterior (VA)	ventral tier	· basal ganglia · cerebellum	cortex area 6
Ventral Posterior Lateral (VPL)	ventral tier	· spinothalamic tract · medial lemniscus	cortex areas 3, 1, 2, (4) (body)
Ventral Posterior Medial (VPM)	ventral tier	trigeminothalamic tracts	cortex areas 3, 1, 2, (4) (face)
Medial Geniculate Body	metathalamic	brachium of inferior colliculus	cortex areas 41, 42 (audition)
Lateral Geniculate Body	metathalamic	optic tract	cortex area 17 (vision)
Association Nuclei			
Medial Dorsal	dorsal tier	· amygdala · temporal lobe	prefrontal cortex
Lateral Dorsal	dorsal tier	numerous areas	cingulate gyrus
Lateral Posterior	dorsal tier	numerous areas	parietal lobe
Pulvinar	dorsal tier	cortex areas 18, 19 (secondary visual)	parietal lobe
Diffuse Nuclei			
Centromedian	intralaminar	brainstem reticular formation	· VPL · VPM · other thalamic nuclei
Subcortical Nuclei			
Reticular	reticular	· frontal lobe	· other thalamic nuclei

zontal section, the internal capsule has a "V" shape, with the point of the V (genu of the internal capsule) directed medially. The anterior limb of the V lies between two components of the basal ganglia, the caudate nucleus anterio-medially, and the lenticular nuclei posteriolaterally. The posterior limb of the V lies lateral to the thalamus (Fig. 10-3). The anterior limb of the internal capsule carries corticopontine fibers from the frontal lobe and thalamic fibers related to anteriorly placed nuclei. The genu of the capsule contains a mixture of thalamic efferent fibers and corticobulbar fibers directed to cranial nerve motor nuclei. The posterior limb of the capsule contains thalamic fibers related to more posteriorly placed nuclei, the fibers of the corticospinal tract, and some additional corticopontine projections. The projecting fibers from the two metathalamic nuclei are not contained in the internal capsule but are carried in specific projection bundles: the auditory radiation that runs slightly ventral to the posterior limb of the capsule, and the optic radiation that forms a posterior boundary for the capsule.

The descending fibers of the internal capsule are collected in the cerebral peduncles essentially maintaining the positions relative to each other that they had in the internal capsule.

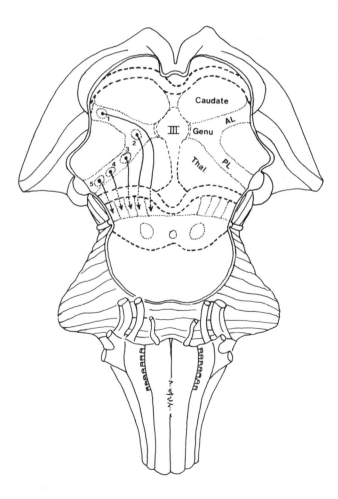

Figure 10-3. Spatial relationships of the internal capsule and cerebral peduncles. The brainstem and diencephalon are presented in a ventral view. The anterior limb *(AL)* of the internal capsule contains frontopontine fibers (1) which come to lie medially in the cerebral peduncles. The genu of the internal capsule contains corticobulbar fibers (2). In the posterior limb *(PL)* of the internal capsule corticospinal fibers for the upper extremity (3) lie anterior to corticospinal fibers for the trunk (not shown), which in turn precede corticospinal fibers for the lower extremity (4). The most posterior fiber group in the posterior limb are the corticopontine fibers (5) which come to lie most laterally and dorsally in the cerebral peduncles.

Review Exercises

10-1.   Structural Models: Several diencephalic models can be generated:
1. Thalamic nuclei (with or without identification of afferent and efferent pathways)
2. Relationships of the corona radiata, internal capsule, cerebral peduncles and corticospinal tracts, with identification of these main components:
   - thalamic projections to the cerebral hemispheres,
   - corticospinal fibers to the upper and lower extremities and the trunk,
   - corticobulbar fibers to the brainstem cranial nerve nuclei,
   - corticopontine fibers to the pontine nuclei.
3. Structures forming the boundaries of the diencephalon.

11

Gating and Sensory Transmission in the Thalamus

The basic processes by which neural information can be modified at synapses have been described earlier (Chap. 4). As a sensory relay station, or synaptic region, the thalamic nuclei are positioned to act as a functional gate between subcortical sensory behavior and cortical perceptual behavior. The gating activity of the thalamus requires extensive reciprocal connections among the brainstem nuclei and pathways, the thalamus, and the cerebral hemispheres. Sensory information up to the level of the thalamus can produce sensorimotor behavior, as has been seen in a discussion of basic spinal reflexes and vestibular reflexes. Sensory information, however, must pass through the thalamus and reach the cerebral cortex before it can become sensory *perception*. Two types of gating activity of the thalamus illustrative of the process of moving from the level of sensation to that of perception are described in this chapter: regulation of states of consciousness and transmission and modification of pain information.

States of Consciousness

Normal consciousness can be divided into two main states, waking and sleeping, with each having several distinct substates. Each state can be characterized by the ability of the cortex to process sensory information, the type of motor behavior shown, and the general homeostatic state of the body. Each state is generated by specific interactions between the brainstem reticular formation, the thalamus, and the cerebral cortex. The neural interactions involved give rise to characteristic patterns of neural electrical activity that can be recorded through the technique of electroencephalography.

Electroencephalography

An electroencephalogram (EEG) is a recording of postsynaptic potentials (not action potentials) in a large collection of cortical neurons. The recording is made typically from either epidural or skin surface (scalp) electrodes. The amplitude of EEG waves is related to the number of active cells and the extent to which they are acting in synchrony. The duration of EEG waves also is related to the extent of synchronous activity and to the duration of the impinging excitatory and inhibitory synaptic events. The frequency of the waves is a function of the frequency of activation of neurons. When there is synchronization there is a lower frequency of EEG waves than when there is desynchronization.

In basic diagnostic electroencephalography, standard configurations of surface electrodes are used. The recording may be either unipolar, in which individual active electrodes are referenced to a bony or cartilagenous portion of the skull, or bipolar, in which pairs of electrodes are referenced to each other (Fig. 11-1).

In addition to recording on-going general activity of cortical cells, the EEG technique may also be used to record evoked potentials that occur in response

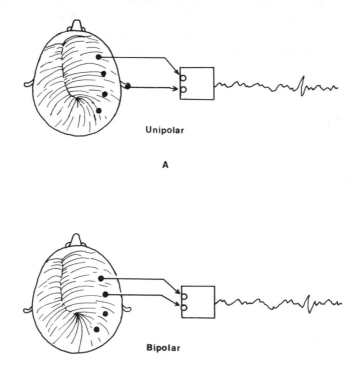

Figure 11-1. Representation of unipolar (A) and bipolar (B) recording arrangements for electroencephalography. Unipolar recording permits localization of a specific signal to a region surrounding the active scalp electrode. Bipolar recording localizes the signal to the region between the two adjacent scalp electrodes. The same evoked potential is illustrated in both recordings.

to specific sensory stimuli (sensory evoked potentials, or SEP). Evoked potential recording has been used experimentally for purposes of localizing cortical regions related to specific sensory, motor, or other behaviors. Clinically, evoked potential recording can be useful particularly for identifying abnormalities in the transmission or cortical processing of specific types of sensory information.

Awake States

During wakefulness, the predominant states of consciousness include the following:
1. Relaxed wakefulness.
2. Arousal.
3. Specific attention.
4. Concentration.

Changing from one awake state to another occurs easily in the normal individual, usually without conscious awareness. Waking states are controlled by activity within the periaqueductal grey of the midbrain that is projected to the thalamus. The thalamic nuclei receiving these projections may include all of the specific relay nuclei, in addition to diffuse nuclei such as the centromedian nucleus. The information in turn is projected widely to the cortex. Generally speaking, in the awake state, thalamocortical activity is desynchronized, and passage of information through the thalamus to the cortex is facilitated.

The *relaxed awake* state is characterized by the following behaviors:
1. Minimal attention to external or internal stimuli.
2. A relaxed posture accompanied by relatively low skeletal muscle tone in all postural muscles.
3. Minimal skeletal motor activity.
4. Closed eyes.

During the relaxed awake state, the predominant EEG waveform is synchronized waves with a frequency of 8 to 13 Hz. These alpha waves can be recorded over the occipital lobes and to a lesser extent over the other lobes. They disappear when the eyes are opened. The synchronization of cortical activity indicated by the alpha waves is produced by a cyclic process involving diffuse and specific relay nuclei of the thalamus and their projection sites in the cerebral cortex. Two types of alpha wave generating processeshave been described: the recruiting response involving the frontal cortex and the augmenting response involving more posterior regions of the cortex, have been described. In the relaxed awake state, the thalamus is open to the transmission of sensory information, but, typically, only minimal information is being transmitted, and there is minimal processing of current sensory information to the level of perception in the cortex. The relaxed awake state can be observed during meditation.

Arousal is the state in which there is generalized awareness of and responsiveness to all stimuli. The eyes are open and there exists a conscious state of expectancy. Motor activity occurs that supports preparation to respond to stimuli that have not yet been specified; there is a generalized increase in postural muscle tone. There is a shift in sympathetic-parasympathetic balance toward sympathetic predominance with increased heart rate, respiratory rate, and blood pressure. Arousal is dependent on activity generated in the ascending reticular activating system (ARAS) of the pons and the mesencephalon. The reticular activity is the result of excitatory input from either the medullary reticular formation or the sensory afferent collateral branches, or both, into the reticular formation throughout the brainstem. Arousal can be generated through conscious cortical commands to a limited extent. During arousal, the EEG shows small amplitude, high-frequency beta waves indicative of generalized desynchronization of activity in the cerebral cortex.

When in the state of *specific attention*, a person is receiving and responding to specific stimuli and blocking reception or attention to all other stimuli. Stimuli other than those being attended to can be perceived only if they are sufficiently novel or important. Motor activity during specific attention serves to enhance reception of the desired stimuli and to perform appropriate responses. Orienting movements of the head, body, and extremities are used to bring the object of attention into optimal relationship to the sensors being used. During the state of specific attention, the EEG shows desynchronization of cortical activity, with the presence of beta waves. Sensory evoked potentials may be superimposed on the beta waves. The SEPs are localized to the area of the cortex that receives the particular sensory information.

Processes involved in generating the state of specific attention include cortical identification of an important stimulus or group of stimuli, followed by selective inhibition of cells of the the reticular nucleus of the thalamus. Inhibition of activity in these cells leads in turn to disinhibition of activity in specific thalamic relay nuclei (Fig. 11-2). As a result of this process, gating of sensory information occurs, with the desired information being passed on through the thalamus to the cortex, and all other information being blocked at the level of the thalamus.

Novel stimuli can break through the generalized thalamic relay inhibition (probably by activating the mesencephalic portion of the ascending reticular activating system), thus shifting the CNS to a state of arousal during which any stimulus may penetrate to the cortex. Specific attention to a repeated stimulus usually decreases through the complex process of habituation. This process appears to be dependent on cortical projections both to the reticular nucleus of the thalamus and to the dorsal horn of the spinal cord. During habituation, stimuli are blocked both at the spinal and the thalamic levels.

During *concentrated mental activity* there is generalized inattention to external stimuli. There tends to be minimal motor activity; activity that does occur tends to be of a stereotyped or automatic nature, with constant repetition (such as repetitive finger movements or chewing a pencil). The predominant EEG wave form may be beta or kappa. Concentration states probably result

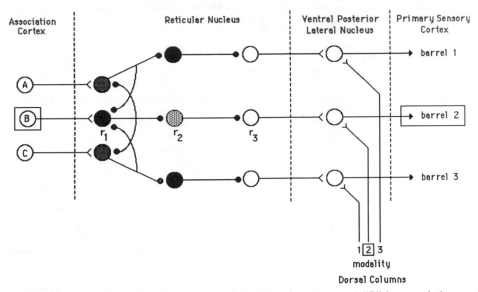

Figure 11-2. Proposed thalamic gating system. Activation of neuron pool "B" in association cortex excites reticular nuclear inhibitory cell group "r-1". Reticular neuron group "r-2" is thus inhibited, and group "r-3" is released from inhibition. The projection of "r-3" into the ventral posterior lateral nucleus (or any other specific relay nucleus) excites its target cell group, facilitating transmission of incoming information (modality 2) through the nucleus and on to its target cortical area (barrel 2). Through the process of surround inhibition originating in the reticular nucleus, transmission of other modalities is simultaneously inhibited. Inhibited inhibitory neurons in all pathways are shaded grey.

from cortical suppression of thalamic relay nucleus activity. Concentration can be changed into a state of arousal by the mediation of novel stimuli.

The awake states so far described have been studied predominantly from the point of view of thalamic handling of sensory information. Since the thalamus also serves as a discriminatory relay point in the generation of motor behavior, there undoubtedly are corresponding descriptions of thalamocortical states under conditions of different types of motor activity.

Sleep

There are two basic types of sleep: *slow wave* sleep (SWS), which has four stages, and paradoxical, or *rapid eye movement* (REM), sleep. These sleep stages can be characterized by differences in EEG pattern, homeostatic state, ease of arousal, motor behavior, and psychological activity (Table 11-1). The changes in CNS behavior marking the transition from the awake state to sleep are probably brought about by changes in reticular system activity. Numerous stimuli or changes in CNS activity have been hypothesized as the cause of the transition from waking to sleeping. Undoubtedly, more than one stimulus or set of associated stimuli is involved. At the onset of sleep, there is decreased activity in the mesencephalic portion of the reticular formation and increased activity in the pontine portion. As a result, there is facilitation of thalamic synchrony that in turn leads to synchronization of cortical activity. This

TABLE 11-1. Characteristics of Sleep Stages

Stage (EEG)	Homeostatic State	Arousal	Motor Behavior	Psychological Activity
SWS				
Stage 1 (alpha waves)	gradually increasing predominance of maintenance activity; slowing of HR, RR; decreasing BP	easy	gradually decreasing spontaneous activity in most muscles combined with gradually increasing tonic activity in some large muscle groups (eg, jaw "jerks")	no specific activity
Stage 2 (alpha spindles)	continuation of stage 1	easy	continuation of stage 1	no specific activity
Stage 3 (slow waves)	continuation of stage 1	difficult	continuation of stage 1	no specific activity
Stage 4 (delta waves)	continuation of stage 1	difficult	phasic activation of of large muscles	night "terrors", sleepwalking superimposed on generalized complete relaxation
REM				
(beta waves)	generalized increase in heart rate, respiratory rate and blood pressure with variability of all homeostatic parameters	very difficult	frequent rapid phasic activation of muscles especially extraocular, ocular, superimposed on general complete relaxation (sleep paralysis)	dreams, nightmares

change in activity can be seen in the alpha wave spindles typical of stage 2 of slow wave sleep. Although the frequency of these waves is the same as that seen in the relaxed awake state, their regular amplitude fluctuations are unique to sleep. One of the possible mechanisms by which alpha spindles could be generated is illustrated in Figure 11-3.

The different types and stages of sleep usually recur in a fairly consistent pattern with each night's sleep (Fig. 11-4). During the first hour of sleep, the person progresses through stages 1-4 of slow wave sleep. Then there is a return to stage 3 or 2, with a period of REM sleep superimposed. Following the REM sleep, there is a return to deeper sleep. This cycle repeats during the night, with the occurrence of stage 3 and 4 sleep becoming less and the periods of REM sleep becoming longer. The person may awake from a final period of REM sleep or from stage 1 of slow wave sleep. When the time available for sleep is shortened, the same sequence of stages occur, but the number of cycles is decreased.

Pain

Pain is a multimodal sensation that typically gives rise to aversive and protective responses and motor behaviors. When pain reaches the level of

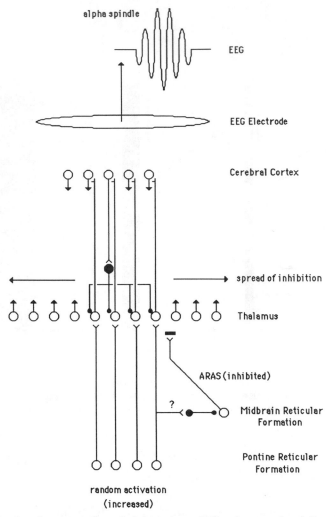

Figure 11-3. Mechanism for generation of alpha wave spindles. Increased activity within the pontine reticular formation excites cell groups within diffuse thalamic nuclei (and may also concurrently inhibit activity within the midbrain reticular formation, transmitted by the ascending reticular activating system—ARAS). The thalamic cells in turn excite cortical cells. Reciprocal projections back to the thalamus pass through inhibitory neurons which simultaneously inhibit a larger group of thalamic cells through divergence. Cells in this larger group regain their excitability at the same time, leading to synchronization of their output in response to the otherwise random reticular input. In turn, a wider group of cortical cells is stimulated simultaneously. The electroencephalogram amplitude reflects the increasing number of synchronous extracellular potentials occurring within a region of cortex over time. As the activated population of cells grows very large, desynchronization occurs as a result of differences in transmission pathway length and random variation in cortical and thalamic cell excitability. There is a corresponding decrease in EMG amplitude.

perception, it usually is associated with negative emotional reactions. Pain can be described in terms of its intensity, modal quality (eg, dull, pricking, burning), duration and persistence, and degree of localization. The *sensation* of pain refers specifically to the activation of discrete (and relatively well-identified) neurons in the PNS and CNS, which generally includes the following:

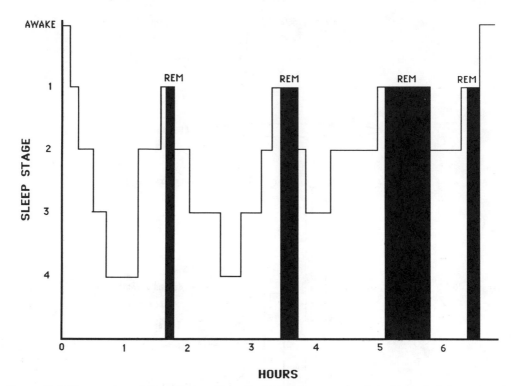

Figure 11-4. Progression of sleep stages. Stage 3 and 4 sleep occurs early in the period. Stage 2 and 1 sleep last longer later during sleep. REM (rapid eye movement) sleep occurs following stage 1 sleep and gradually increases in duration during the period of sleep.

1. Peripheral nociceptors and their afferent fibers.
2. Second order afferents within the dorsal horn of the spinal cord or the spinal nucleus of cranial nerve V.
3. Ascending pathways to the thalamus and the brainstem reticular system.
4. Pain-specific neurons in various thalamic nuclei.

Note that as described here, pain *sensation* does not involve activation of any cerebral cortical structures; therefore, pain sensation does not imply any conscious awareness of a pain stimulus. Given just the substrate described so far, appropriate and fairly complex motor responses to pain stimuli can be generated by involuntary or reflex motor pathways.

Normally, the sensation of pain is linked with the perception of pain. Pain perception requires, at a minimum, appropriate activation of thalamic cells, projection to the sensory and limbic regions of the cerebral cortex, and appropriate activation of cells in these cortical regions. By dissociating the thalamic activity from the cortex, pain sensation can occur without pain perception. As will be discussed later, pain perception can occur without normal pain sensation activity in certain circumstances.

Anatomical Substrate for Pain (Fig. 11-5)

Noxious, or painful, stimuli include any stimuli that potentially or actually damage tissue. Such stimuli may be mechanical, thermal, chemical, or electromagnetic in nature. Nociceptors are found in all tissues and organs, with the exception of the neural and glial tissue of the CNS. (Nociceptors, however, are found in the meninges and in the walls of blood vessels supplying the CNS.) Nociceptors are either free nerve endings or receptors, with a minimal capsule, that are innervated by C and A-delta (or group IV and III) afferent fibers. Given the range of diameter and myelination of fibers innervating nociceptors, one would expect a corresponding range in conduction velocity, with C fibers (group IV) conducting at 0.5-2 m/sec and the A-delta (group III) fibers conducting approximately 10 times faster. This dichotomy of conduction velocity for pain information has been suggested as one cause of the perception of "dual" pain following a single noxious stimulus. Not all nociceptors respond to each type of noxious stimulus, providing the possibility for discrimination of pain quality at the level of the nociceptor. The transduction process for nociceptors is still unclear: in some cases it obviously involves

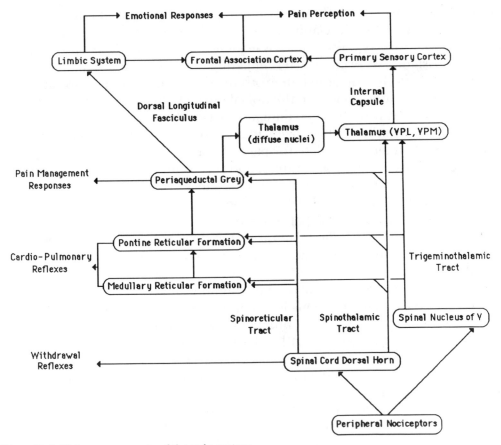

Figure 11-5. Major components of the pain system.

chemical alteration of electrical properties of the receptor membrane; but in other cases the electrical properties may be altered by direct mechanical deformation of the terminal. There is also the possibility that transduction is the result of the release, from damaged cells, of specific neurotransmitter chemicals such as bradykinin, histamine, prostaglandins, and substance P.

Current knowledge indicates that all peripheral nociceptive neurons in spinal nerves synapse with second order neurons within the spinal dorsal horn or intermediate region. Analogous connections are made for nociceptors in the face projecting to the spinal nucleus of cranial nerve V. Fibers entering the cord may ascend a short distance in Lissauer's tract just outside the marginal zone. It appears that most unmyelinated nociceptive fibers enter the dorsal horn from its dorsomedial aspect and synapse in laminae I and II (marginal zone and substantia gelatinosa). There is additional evidence for nociceptive fiber synapses, particularly in lamina V and lamina X. Additional terminals are scattered throughout the dorsal horn. Some of the connections, particularly in laminae I, II, and X, are modality-specific; many others are multimodal. A good correlation exists between identified synaptic regions and areas from which spinothalamic and spinoreticular tract fibers arise. It seems likely that a correlation exists between different types of nociceptors, different synapse locations, and different ascending fibers with specific terminal locations, but details of such relationships have not yet been worked out. At many of the dorsal horn synapses, there is evidence of axoaxonic synapses supporting the possibility of primary afferent gating at this level in the pain pathway.

At least 8 to 10 suggested neurotransmitters have been associated with known pain synaptic regions in the dorsal horn. These include both excitatory and inhibitory transmitters. To date, no specific "pain-transmitting" or "pain-inhibiting" transmitters have been identified with complete certainty. Substance P is one major candidate for pain-transmitting activity; the enkephalins and endorphins (opiate transmitters) and serotonin are strong candidates for pain-inhibiting transmitters. Other transmitters are certainly involved in the complex synaptic circuitry of the dorsal horn.

The two main ascending pathways for pain information are the crossed spinothalamic tract and the bilateral spinoreticular tract. The spinothalamic tract contains both rapidly and slowly conducting fibers that have synapses mainly in the ventral posterior nuclei of the thalamus. These fibers send collaterals to the reticular formation throughout the brainstem. The spinoreticular fibers terminate at various levels in the reticular formation; from there, polysynaptic projections go to a number of thalamic nuclei. These projections are probably (but not certainly) less location- and modality-specific than the spinothalamic projections. Projections from the periaqueductal grey also bypass the thalamus to have synapses directly with portions of the limbic system. Within the thalamus, synaptic contact is made either with cells that are pain-specific, as may be the case in the ventroposterior nuclei or with multimodal cells. Cortical cells receiving pain projections from the thalamus may be clustered in modality-specific primary sensory areas of the parietal lobe.

There is some indication that pain-specific cortical cells exist, but the nearly universal lack of pain perception following direct electrical stimulation of the sensory cortex suggests either that the cells are multimodal or that they only code for pain when stimulated with a specific input pattern that is difficult to mimic experimentally.

Neurophysiological Coding For Pain

Starting at the level of the nociceptor, it is evident that the production of pain sensation is dependent not only on activating appropriate neurons (location coding) but also on activating them in a pattern that codes for pain. For example, frequency of stimulation of nociceptors and of action potential transmission in primary afferents can make the difference between a painful or a nonpainful sensation. Within the spinal cord, the possibility for modulation of pain sensation is increased both through presynaptic inhibition and postsynaptic inhibition of multimodal cells. Melzack and Wall's "gate" theory of pain was based on the observation that concurrent activation of large diameter, low threshold, primary afferents could block transmission of pain information through either of these two types of inhibition.

At the thalamic level, there is definite evidence that pain, like at least some other sensory modalities, is dependent on appropriately timed activation of either unimodal (pain-specific) or polymodal thalamic cells. The transmission of such a code to the sensory cortex may also be necessary for pain perception. It has been suggested that a "pain" code could be developed by reciprocal excitation between specific cells in the ventral lateral nuclei and polymodal cells in the diffuse nuclei of the thalamus. A general scheme for developing a pain code by this mechanism is outlined in Figure 11-6. The mechanism depends not only on reciprocal thalamic connections but also on correctly timed multiple inputs from various ascending pathways. With this type of code, which is very dependent on action potential interval timing, code disruption and thus pain modulation could occur fairly easily, arising from a number of sources.

Pain Modulation

Pain sensation and perception potentially can be modulated at any level of the neuraxis at which synapses in ascending pain pathways are located. The basic mechanisms involved are either block of transmission of pain information or alteration of the pattern of activity. Transmission block by simple presynaptic or postsynaptic inhibition probably occurs at the level of the dorsal horn; code disruption probably occurs in the thalamus. Some of the possible modulatory pathways and their interactions are outlined in Figure 11-7.

From an examination of Figure 11-7, it is evident that the periaqueductal grey can play an important role in pain modulation, as can large diameter primary afferents. There is growing evidence that the periaqueductal grey demonstrates somatotopic organization. Convergent projections from large

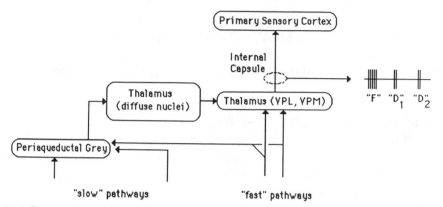

Figure 11-6. Proposed mechanism for developing a thalamic frequency code for pain. Rapidly projecting pathways to specific thalamic relay nuclei (VPL, VPM) produce an initial high-frequency burst ("F")
of activity which is sent to the primary sensory cortex. Delayed activity ("D-1") occurs as a result of
slower pathway projections through the reticular formation (periaqueductal grey) and diffuse thalamic
nuclei. Still later activity ("D-2") may be generated in response to reciprocal activity within the involved
thalamic nuclei. The precise timing of the late bursts of activity is probably important in coding for
sensory modality—in this case, pain.

diameter primary afferent pathways to specific parts of the periaqueductal
grey may be the basis for modulation of pain in one part of the body through
nonnociceptive stimulation in another region. Descending pain sensation
modulation initiated from the periaqueductal grey is transmitted through
reticulospinal pathways with their origin in various raphe nuclei, particularly
the nucleus raphe magnus of the pons. The transmission pathways involve
opiate neurotransmitters between the periaqueductal grey and the raphe
nuclei and involve serotonin between the raphe nuclei and the spinal dorsal
horn. Within the dorsal horn itself, a number of transmitters may be involved
including, again, those in the opiate group. Ascending pain perception modulation from the periaqueductal grey appears to be dependent on distortion or
interruption of the frequency coding of pain signals in the thalamus.

Pain perception and sensation can also be modified through direct cortical
intervention at spinal and thalamic levels using either corticothalamic pathways that alter the state of arousal or attention or indirect corticospinal
pathways. Various physical therapeutic techniques for modifying pain and the
probable mechanisms through which they and other pain intervention techniques act are summarized in Table 11-2.

Pathophysiological Pain

Under certain circumstances, pain can exist without providing its normal
protective function. In some cases a real noxious stimulus is the basis for such
pain; in others, many functional aspects of pain sensation are absent but pain
perception persists.

Sympathetic reflex dystrophy is an example of a positive feedback loop
causing persistent pain. A specific initial stimulus, usually but not always

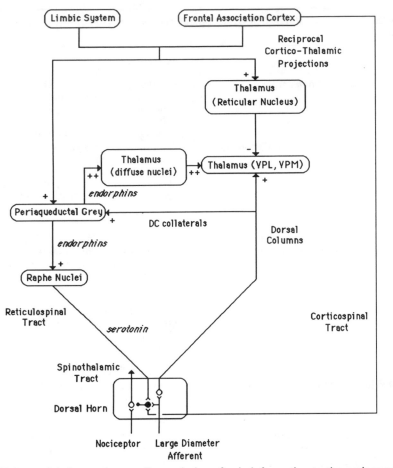

Figure 11-7. Pain modulation pathways. Transmission of pain information to the periaqueductal grey can lead to endorphin release. The endorphins are transmitted both to the raphe nuclei and to the diffuse thalamic nuclei. Activity in the raphe nuclei projects to the spinal dorsal horn (or spinal nucleus of the Vth nerve) using serotonin as the neurotransmitter. Both of these actions can suppress transmission of pain information. Activation of large diameter afferents can cause block of pain information transmission both by gating in the dorsal horn and by activation of the periaqueductal grey. Transmission of pain information from the thalamus can be blocked through the action of endorphins from the periaqueductal grey or through gating activity probably mediated by the reticular nucleus of the thalamus. Additionally, cortical activity can be transmitted to the dorsal horn to assist in gating pain transmission there.

noxious, causes excitation of sympathetic preganglionic or postganglionic cells. Activation of these neurons leads to persistent vasoconstriction and subsequent trophic changes in tissue. Additionally, activation of sensory fibers in the autonomic system may result in release of pain-inducing chemicals at the peripheral terminals of these fibers, providing another route for positive feedback. These effects can generate persistent intrinsic noxious stimulation that can continue the cycle indefinitely, even in the absence of renewed extraneous noxious stimulation. Similar positive feedback pain cycles, not

TABLE 11-2. Summary of Neurophysiological Bases for Therapeutic Pain Intervention Techniques

Mechanism	Techniques
Transmission blockade of nociceptors	· electrical stimulation of small diameter afferents (high frequency, low intensity) · local anesthetics acting on small diameter afferents · section of the dorsal horn or dorsal root
Spinal PAD by direct large diameter afferents (eg, rubbing the skin)	· natural stimulation of large diameter afferent axoaxonic synapse activity · transcutaneous electrical nerve stimulation (TENS) (low frequency, high intensity) · acupuncture and derivative techniques
Spinal postsynaptic inhibition from large diameter afferents	· same techniques which produce spinal PAD
Transmission blockade in the spinal cord	· tractotomy of the spinothalamic tract
Disruption of pain code in the thalamus	· natural stimulation of large diameter afferents · TENS (various frequencies and intensities) · acupuncture and derivative techniques · dorsal column stimulation with implanted electrodes · PAG stimulation with implanted electrodes · stimulation of diffuse thalamic nuclei with implanted electrodes · systemic opiate administration · ablation of diffuse thalamic nuclei · ablation of ventral posterior nuclei
Decreased excitability of ventral posterior thalamic nuclei	· systemic administration of narcotics or general anesthetics · cortical inhibition by hypnosis, biofeedback or behavior modification
Transmission blockade to the cortex	· selective lesioning of the ventral posterior nucleus or its projections
Descending spinal dorsal horn inhibition from the raphe nuclei	· TENS (various frequencies and intensities) · acupuncture and derivative techniques · systemic opiate administration

necessarily involving the sympathetic nerves, occur in painful skeletal muscle and joint tissue. In this case, reflex protective muscle contraction (splinting) intended to eliminate one source of pain can lead to oxygen deprivation in the active muscle, thereby providing a new pain stimulus. Such pain cycles are best treated by breaking the transmission of pain information at some point.

Thalamic, or deafferentiation, pain, sometimes called dysesthesia, is persistent, recurrent pain occurring in the absence of any identifiable noxious stimulation. Dysesthesia is associated frequently with amputation, spinal cord injury, peripheral nerve injury, trigeminal neuralgia, and the sequelae of herpes zoster (shingles) infections. This type of pain essentially originates at the thalamic level, with two possible mechanisms being as follows:

1. Release of the PAG from normal dorsal column input, giving rise to more synchronous input to diffuse thalamic nuclei sufficient to generate pain code activity.

2. Increase of ventral posterior nucleus excitability through deafferentia-
    tion hyperexcitability.

Dyesthesias usually develop over time; thus they are examples of "learned"
behavior and, as such, may represent synaptic changes. Thalamic pain is
particularly difficult to treat effectively because of the level of the neuraxis at
which it occurs. Therapies directed at altering spinal pain activity or transmission are not usually effective. The generation of the pain code can be altered
by periaqueductal grey stimulation through implanted electrodes or by the
systemic administration of opiates, the former being technically more difficult
but having far fewer negative side effects. Stimulation of the dorsal columns,
if those ascending pathways are intact, may also be effective. Selective lesion-
ing of the thalamus or its cortical projections has been used in some cases, but
this approach has obvious disadvantages in that it removes all sense modalities
for a given part of the body. The least invasive approach is the use of hypnosis
and behavior modification, to decrease pain perception.

Chronic pain perception resulting from an initial noxious stimulus that is
subsequently removed is most difficult to treat and usually requires a very
thorough evaluation to determine the possible etiology of the perceived pain
and the presence, if any, of actual pain sensation activity. Frequently, physical
and psychological therapeutic approaches are more effective in managing
chronic pain than are invasive treatments aimed at removing a source of pain.

Referred Pain

As a result of nociceptive primary afferents converging in the lower laminae of the dorsal horn, stimulation of nociceptors in different anatomical
locations may produce pain perception that is localized, or referred, to a site
distant from the actual point of stimulation. Pain stimulus location referral is
noted primarily with stimulation of viscera, indicating that there is frequent
convergence of visceral nociceptors on dorsal horn cells that also receive
nondiscrete sensory input of various modalities from muscle or skin receptors.
Localization of referred pain is typically diffuse rather than specific. Patterns
of convergence, however, are very specific, permitting diagnostic localization
of the source of referred pain on the basis of the area of referral and the
quality of the pain perceived.

Review Exercises

11-1. You are to treat a patient who complains of lower back pain which has
persisted for ten days.
- What pain modulation techniques could you try which would selectively
  cause inhibition of pain transmission at the level of the spinal cord?
  Describe the neurophysiological mechanisms involved in each type of
  treatment.
- If non-invasive treatment proves ineffective in decreasing the patient's
  pain, what types of surgical interventions could be tried to inhibit trans-

mission of pain sensation to the level of the cerebral cortex? On the basis of what you know about pain transmission pathways, select one intervention site and technique which would be most likely to decrease pain sensation (or perception). Justify your choice.

11-2.   On the basis of your knowledge of the role of the brainstem reticular formation in controlling states of consciousness, what state(s) would you expect to see in an individual (or experimental animal) with transection of the neuraxis between the midbrain and the thalamus? Would such a condition permit perception of any stimuli? If so, what modalities would be perceived? Would the person or animal be able to demonstrate any somatic or autonomic motor responses indicating the existence of perception of stimuli? If so, identify these responses and describe the pathways making them possible.

The pathological state of coma can be caused by, among other things, compression of the midbrain with concomitant loss of activity of various midbrain cell bodies and fibers. There is growing evidence that for at least some persons in coma perception and memory of at least some sensory stimuli is possible. Would your responses to the questions concerning neuraxis transection provide hypotheses to support these observations?

12

Cerebral Hemisphere Gross Anatomy and Cytoarchitecture

Historically, there have been three major theories concerning the relationship between cerebral cortical structure and cortical function. Two theories developed separately during the nineteenth century: the localization theory and the aggregate field theory. Both were attempts to explain the increasing amounts of complex anatomical and psychological information related to cortical function. The localization theory suggested that specific psychological functions could be assigned to regions of the cerebral hemispheres operating independently of each other. The theory was based primarily on observations of specific types of psychological dysfunctions clearly related to alterations in brain structure seen at autopsy. The theory was popularized as "phrenology," by Gall and Spurzheim. According to the phrenologists, growth of specific regions of the hemispheres indicated either a strong potential for or the presence of the psychological function supposedly localized to the region. The function-specific growth of the hemispheres was reflected presumably in the development of "bumps" in the overlying bone, which could be palpated. Phrenological examination by palpation of an individual's skull was accepted widely in nonprofessional circles as a means of determining the strengths and weaknesses of a person's character. As indicated in Figure 12-1, the psychological characteristics that could be analyzed by this method very strongly reflected the prevailing values of the society in which the theory was developed. Phrenology, particularly the practice of judging character by the bumps on a person's head, fell into disrepute by the turn of the century. The basic localization theory from which phrenology developed, however, is still a valid expression of what is currently known about the ability of different regions of the hemispheres to control specific functions.

The second theory of cortical function to develop during the nineteenth

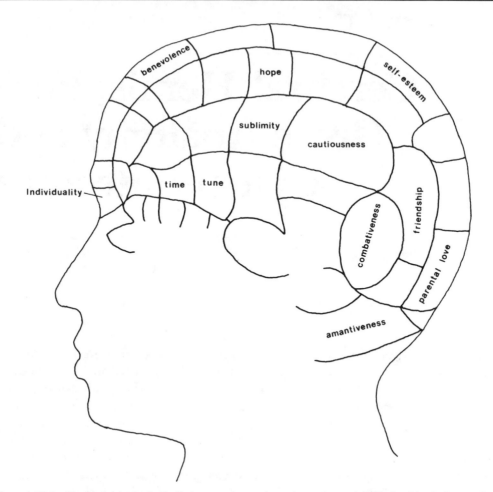

Figure 12-1. Phrenological skull. Only certain regions have been labelled with their ascribed characteristics.

century was the aggregate field theory. It was first stated by Flourens in the early part of the century and was still supported by various neuroscientists such as Head in England, Goldstein in Germany, and Lashley in the United States, until the middle of the current century. In opposition to the localization theory, this theory suggested that all cortical functions were dependent on the integrated and cooperative activity of the entire cerebral cortex. The theory was supported by various experiments aimed at discovering precise locations for complex psychological functions. The inability to discover such localization, coupled with the observation that many psychological functions deteriorated gradually as the amount of hemisphere was nonspecifically decreased by ablation, suggested to researchers that precise localization, at least for complex functions, was not as important as interconnections among widespread parts of the hemispheres.

The currently accepted theory of cortical hemispheric function is the cellular connection theory that incorporates the clearly supported aspects of both of these earlier theories. All hemispheric functions are suggested to be dependent on discrete and identifiable collections of cells that act through integrated, specific connections with other related cell groups both within the hemispheres and in other parts of the neuraxis. The clinical studies that particularly initiated this theory include the studies on epilepsy by Hughlings Jackson and Wilder Penfield and the studies of language function by Paul Broca and Carl Wernicke during the early part of this century. More recent structural and functional observations strongly support this theory.

The anatomical bases for the cellular connection theory are primarily 1) evidence of discrete regions of the hemisphere in which the cytoarchitecture and cell morphology is distinctly different from that seen in other regions and 2) evidence of specific patterns of interconnecting fibers intrinsic and extrinsic to the hemispheres. The cortex of the cerebral hemispheres is composed of three main types: paleocortex in portions of the temporal lobe, archicortex in the hippocampus, and neocortex in the remainder of the hemispheres. Paleocortex and archicortex are three layered. The basic six-layered arrangement of the neocortex differs from one location to the other as a result of differing concentrations of various types of cells and their fiber connections. The neocortex of the cerebral hemispheres can basically be subdivided into three functional types of regions: motor, sensory, and association (Fig. 12-2). Motor cortex is located in the frontal lobe; sensory cortex in the parietal, temporal and occipital lobes; and association cortex in the frontal, temporal and parietal lobes. The cytoarchitecture of the neocortex shows significant variation in and among these three major functional regions. The precise cell morphology within each cell layer, the types of synaptic connections, and thus the arrangement of fibers and even the existence of certain layers is variable from one cortical region to another. This cytoarchitectural variability has been used by a number of authors in establishing classification systems for cortical regions. The best known of these systems is probably the one developed by Brodmann (Fig. 12-3).

The six layers of the neocortex contain basically two types of cells: stellate cells having axonal projections that remain primarily in the cortical region in which the cell body is situated and pyramidal cells having axons that project out from the cortical region to other regions of the neocortex or the neuraxis. Stellate cells have dendrites confined either to the layer in which the cell body is located or to the layers immediately adjacent. Stellate cell axons make contact with the dendrites of pyramidal cells and other stellate cells in specific patterns (Fig. 12-4). *Horizontal* (S_h) stellate cell axons make multiple connections on dendrites of pyramidal and other stellate cells within the cell layer containing the cell body. *Climbing* (S_c) stellate cell axons make multiple contacts with the radially directed apical dendrites of pyramidal cells. *Basket* (B) stellate cells make contact with the cell bodies of pyramidal and other stellate cells, either within or beyond the layer in which the basket cell body is contained. The basket cells in particular are inhibitory in function, with

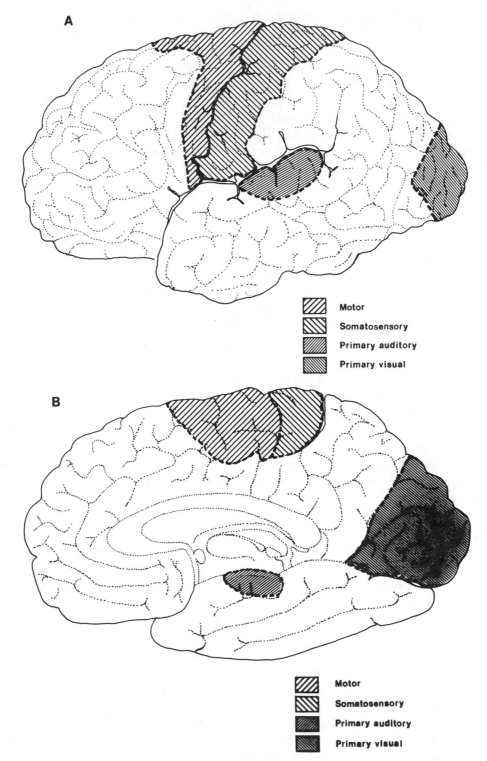

Figure 12-2. Major functional divisions of the cerebral hemispheres. A: lateral view. B: Mid-sagittal view. Unshaded regions have predominantly association or integration functions.

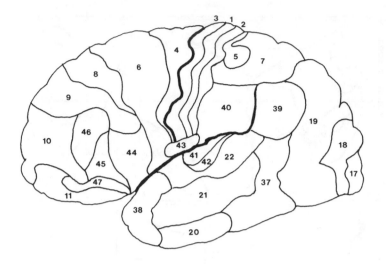

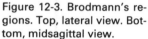

Figure 12-3. Brodmann's regions. Top, lateral view. Bottom, midsagittal view.

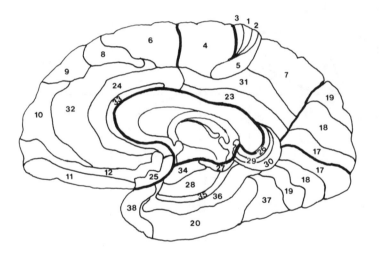

synapses positioned in locations that can very directly control transmission by way of pyramidal cells. Stellate cell bodies may be found in all cell layers, but are in particularly high concentration in layers II, III, IV, and VI. Pyramidal cells are so named from the shape of their cell bodies. They have two sets of dendrites: a major apical dendrite that projects radially outward from the cell body, and branches in more outwardly placed cell layers and a set of basal dendrites that lie in the layer of the cell body or the immediately adjacent inner layer. Pyramidal cell bodies are located in layers II , III, V, and VI. Their axons, in all cases, project out of the cortex. Projections from layer II and III pyramidal cells are directed to other regions of the cortex. Layer V pyramidal cells project to a variety of subcortical structures; layer VI pyramidal cells project to the thalamus (Fig. 12-5).

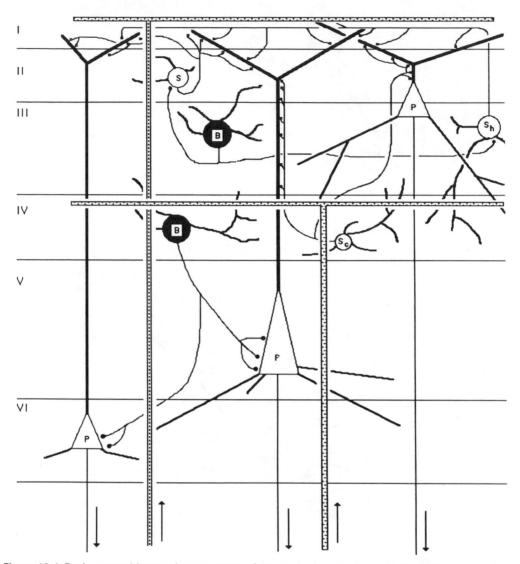

Figure 12-4. Basic cytoarchitectural components of the cerebral cortex. Layer I is the outermost cortical layer. Primary cellular components include 1) cells with projections within the cortex: basket cells (B), stellate cells (S), climbing stellate cells (S$_c$) and horizontal stellate cells (S$_h$) and 2) pyramidal cells (P) which project out of the cortex. Cortical afferent fibers branch predominantly in layers I and IV.

Early cytoarchitectural studies in which synaptic connections and branching patterns of axons and dendrites were examined indicated that the neocortex was not organized as an extensive network but rather as a collection of relatively discrete, radially-oriented cell columns, now called barrels (Fig. 12-6). These barrels may be defined anatomically by either common points of origin for incoming axons or common points of destination for outgoing axons from pyramidal cells, or both. There now is considerable evidence that barrels have a functional, as well as a structural identity; that is, any given

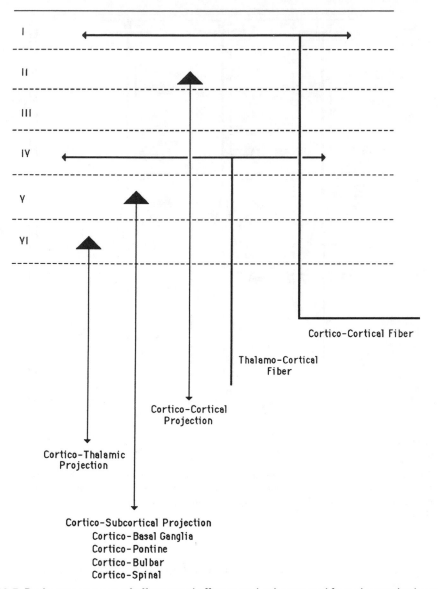

Figure 12-5. Basic arrangement of afferent and efferent projections to and from the cerebral cortex.

barrel or set of barrels has a particular and rather limited set of functions it can perform. There is also growing evidence that the organization of the neocortex into barrels is a dynamic state that can change over time and that to a very large extent is under the influence of input from places such as the brainstem reticular formation and the limbic system. This dynamic organization of barrels has been linked to changes in behavior described as learning. The functional architecture of barrels has been shown to be altered by changes in the amount of use of the sensory or motor function related to the

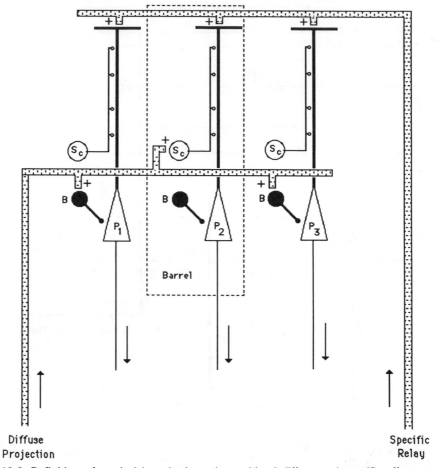

Diffuse
Projection

Specific
Relay

Figure 12-6. Definition of cortical barrels through combined diffuse and specific afferent synaptic arrangements. Surround inhibition involving climbing stellate cells and inhibitory basket cells defines a barrel with specific functions. The synaptic connections illustrated for the afferent fibers is open to modification.

barrel, the amount of attention given to that function, and the affective quality of that attention.

A number of possible fiber connections support the function of individual cortical regions. These can be generally classed as follows:

1. Local projection fibers (layer II-III pyramidal cells): short axons connecting cells within a barrel or in adjacent, functionally similar barrels.
2. Short association fibers (layer II-III pyramidal cells): axons forming connections among adjacent groups of barrels with related functions, such as between barrels in the precentral and postcentral gyrus.
3. Long association fibers (layer II-III pyramidal cells): axons forming connections among anatomically distant but functionally related regions of the neocortex.
4. Commissural fibers (layer II-III pyramidal cells): axons forming connec-

tions among functionally related regions in the two hemispheres.

5. Projection fibers (layers V and VI pyramidal cells): axons projecting from the neocortex to lower regions of the neuraxis.

6. Afferent fibers: axons entering a region of the neocortex and originating either within the cortex (one of the types listed above) or in other locations of the neuraxis (cortical afferents).

Of these fiber types, a number are easily identifiable on dissection. Short association fibers form the layer of white matter immediately underlying all of the hemispheric gyri. Long association fibers are located more deeply in the white matter and make up the following major fasciculi (Fig. 12-7):

1. Superior longitudinal fasciculus connecting frontal, parietal, and occipital lobes.

2. Arcuate fasciculus connecting temporal, parietal, and frontal lobes and carrying primarily language information.

3. Inferior longitudinal fasciculus connecting the temporal and parietal lobes.

4. Frontooccipital fasciculus connecting the frontal and occipital lobes inferiorly through the temporal lobe.

5. Uncinate fasciculus connecting the frontal and temporal lobes anteriorly.

All neocortical commissural fibers run in the corpus callosum. Additional

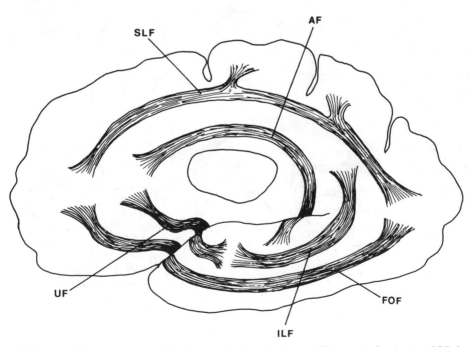

Figure 12-7. Long fiber pathways within the cerebral hemispheres. *AF,* arcuate fasciculus; *FOF,* frontooccipital fasciculus; *ILF,* inferior longitudinal fasciculus; *SLF,* superior longitudinal fasciculus; *UF,* uncinate fasciculus.

commissures visible in the cerebral hemispheres, the fornix, the anterior commissure, the posterior commissure, and the habenular commissure, all connect either rhinencephalic (limbic, paleocortex and archicortex) structures or portions of the diencephalon (Fig. 12-8).

Axons entering the cortex make connection with cell bodies and dendrites in specific patterns within the cortical layers. Layer I primarily receives axons projecting from other regions of the cortex. Layer IV is the major reception layer for projections from the thalamus (Fig. 12-5).

Somatic Sensory-Motor Cortex

The somatic sensorimotor cortex includes basically Brodmann areas 6 and 4 for motor cortex and areas 3a, 3b, 1, and 2 for sensory cortex. Area 6 is subdivided typically into a lateral premotor area and a medial supplementary motor area. Area 4 is called the primary motor cortex. Areas 3, 1, and 2, ranging from anterior to posterior, make up the primary somatosensory (S-I) cortex. The part of these areas adjacent to the Sylvian fissure and more posterior in the parietal lobe (area 5) is termed the secondary somatosensory (S-II) cortex. Within the somatic sensorimotor cortex, barrels are organized both by modality (or, more generally, source of afferent fibers) and by somatotopy. The somatotopic organization is most evident in the primary motor cortex (area 4; precentral gyrus) and the primary sensory cortex (areas 3a, 3b,

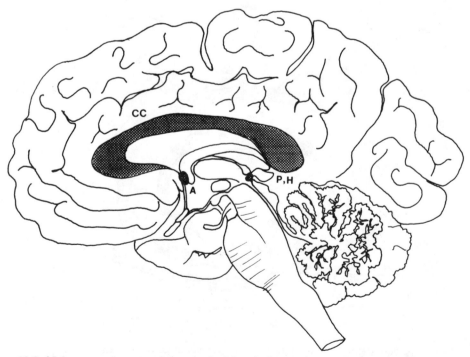

Figure 12-8. Major commissures of the cerebral hemispheres. *A,* anterior commissure; *CC,* corpus collosum; *H,* habenular commissure; *P,* posterior commissure.

1, and 2; postcentral gyrus). Areas 4, 3, 1, 2, and 5 receive direct sensory input by way of thalamocortical projections from the ventroposterior thalamus (VPL, VPM), with area 4 receiving much less input than the sensory cortex. A very close topographic correlation exists between primary sensory and motor areas; it is supported by short, direct corticocortical association fibers crossing under the central sulcus. The input to the sensory cortex can subsequently be projected to association regions for further hierarchical processing, or projected to motor cortex for regulation of activity in motor pyramidal cells (Fig. 12-9).

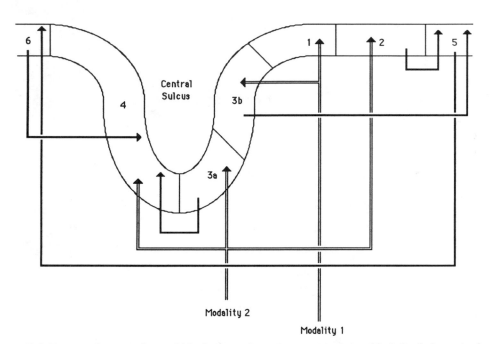

Figure 12-9. Pattern of connections within the somatic sensory motor cortex. Modality 1 shows typical projections for proprioceptors; modality 2 shows projections for skin sensory receptors. The actual mosaic of modality projection within cytoarchitectural areas is considerably more complex than that illustrated. Sequential cortico-cortical processing of sensory information among areas is essential for integration and modification of individual bits of sensory information with other sensory modalities and with information from association cortex. Direct proprioceptor projections to area 4 are probably the substrate for long loop stretch reflexes.

Review Exercises

12-1.   Choose one sensory modality or sub-modality and describe how you would design afferent sensory pathways which could project this information effectively to a brain (cerebral cortex) which was organized strictly on the basis of isolated, localized functional units. In what ways would your design differ from that you are already aware of for sensory afferent pathways?

12-2. Structural Models

1 It is possible to make in situ dissections of the long intrahemispheric fiber pathways. Consider making such a dissection or making a model of these pathways.

2. Make a three-dimensional model of a cortical barrel, indicating the synaptic connections which determine its boundaries. In various regions of the cortex barrels may have cross-sectional shapes varying from roughly circular, to extended ovals with irregular outlines.

13

Motor Control Systems

Motor system components can be grouped functionally into higher, middle, and lower levels (Fig. 13-1). The higher level consists of the limbic system and portions of association cortex located primarily in the frontal and parietal lobes. The middle level includes the sensorimotor cortex, the cerebellum with its associated brainstem nuclei (red nucleus and inferior olivary nuclear complex), and the basal ganglia. The lower level includes the reticular formation in the brainstem and various motor nuclei with their associated interneurons in the brainstem and spinal cord. The primary function of the higher level is to develop goals for motor activity. The middle level components are involved in learning and activating strategies to achieve those goals; the lower level sets background levels of motor neuron excitability and carries out the commands directed to it from the middle level. Motor activity at all times is dependent on both sensory information and internal reference copies of system state information about what each level is currently doing (Fig. 13-2).

Goal setting by the limbic system and prefrontal and parietal association cortex may occur either on the basis of current sensory information or as a result of prior information held in memory and combined with current information. The current emotional state, the need to maintain homeostasis, and cognitive information also are taken into consideration in setting motor goals.

In the middle level of the motor hierarchy, each component has major responsibilities: the sensorimotor cortex generates motor command patterns that are always associated with sensory and system state modulatory programs. The cerebellum is responsible for establishing the timing of activation of cells either in the brainstem and spinal cord or in the sensorimotor cortex. The basal ganglia primarily adjust motor commands to make them spatially appropriate (scaling of movements). Together, these components have a major responsibility for setting appropriate movement trajectories and recruitment patterns for muscles and motor units. Movement trajectories are the path each involved joint takes in moving the body or body parts. For any desired movement, a very large number of possible trajectories are available; it is the

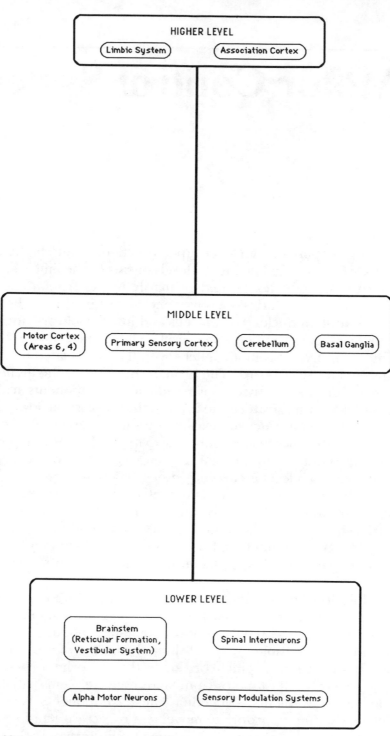

Figure 13-1. Motor system hierarchy.

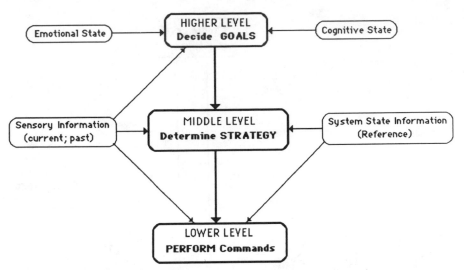

Figure 13-2. Primary information transmission paths within the motor hierarchy.

responsibility of the middle level to select the most effective trajectory. Patterns of muscle activation involve selection of muscles, determination of the timing of muscle activation, and determination of motor unit recruitment patterns within individual muscles. A discussion of functional muscle activation patterns is properly in the realm of kinesiology. Again, there are many different activation patterns that could achieve a particular goal; the middle level selects among them.

In the lower level, there are two subdivisions: the brainstem nuclei and the reticular formation and spinal interneuron systems, and the final common path of the alpha motor neurons. The brainstem nuclei, in particular the vestibular nuclei, and the brainstem reticular formation along with the interneurons of the spinal cord, are involved primarily in adjusting and maintaining levels of alpha motor neuron excitability. The alpha motor neurons then remain as the final command path for enacting the decisions made by all higher levels.

The probability that an action potential will be generated in any given alpha motor neuron or set of alpha motor neurons is dependent on the balance of excitatory and inhibitory synaptic activity impinging on the neuron(s). The possible synaptic contacts with alpha motor neurons include direct sensory contacts, direct contacts from descending motor control pathways, recurrent contacts from Renshaw cells, and indirect contacts from sensory or motor control systems through spinal interneurons (Fig. 13-3). Direct sensory and descending motor control synapses are predominantly if not exclusively excitatory. Renshaw cells, of course, are inhibitory. The spinal interneurons may provide either excitation or inhibition. In addition to variation in polarity, the

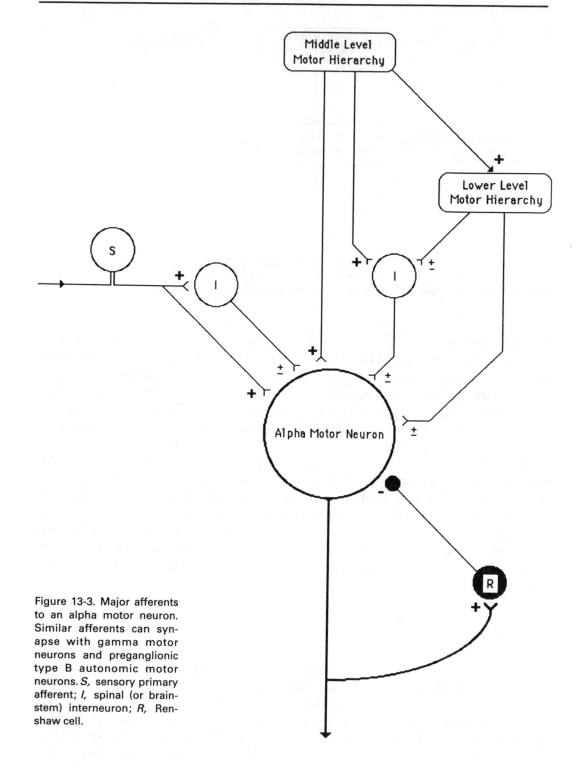

Figure 13-3. Major afferents to an alpha motor neuron. Similar afferents can synapse with gamma motor neurons and preganglionic type B autonomic motor neurons. *S,* sensory primary afferent; *I,* spinal (or brainstem) interneuron; *R,* Renshaw cell.

synaptic input to alpha motor neurons can vary in its time characteristics so that some inputs can be described as tonic and others as phasic. The time characteristics of the synapse activity is not always fixed for a given type of input. A final factor that must be considered is the strength or security of the synaptic contact. As an example, the monosynaptic stretch reflex pathway described in Chapter 7 has a high level of security of synaptic contact with homonymous alpha motorneurons and a decreasing level of security with functionally more distant (synergistic) alpha motorneurons. The systems typically used to adjust the tonic background level of excitation of alpha motor neurons are the brainstem motor control centers (vestibular system and reticular formation), the spinal interneurons, and to a limited extent, the sensory input. Examples of the gross changes in alpha motor neuron excitability that can be brought about by these systems will be discussed below (postural maintenance). Sensory input and most of the descending motor control systems can provide phasic changes in excitability on the basis of this background. Because sensory input can have an effect on alpha motor neuron excitability, modulation of sensory activity by descending systems in close correlation with commands to alpha motor neurons is an important part of producing appropriate muscle activation.

Under normal circumstances, the range of level of excitation of alpha motor neurons is normally quite large. When various controlling components are either removed from the system or released from inhibition as a result of pathological changes in the nervous system, the possible levels of excitation can become quite limited. Clinically, the level of excitability of alpha motor neurons (or the probability of production of an action potential) has been evaluated by measuring the muscle contraction response to various sensory inputs (eg, tendon tap, passive movement of a joint at varying velocities, alterations of body or limb position). The motor behavior elicited is called *tone*. Again, with a normal CNS, muscle tone can be quite varied; it appropriately supports whatever type of passive or active use of muscles is occurring. With neural pathology, the muscle response to manipulation becomes limited or stereotyped; it may be described as an excess of tone or activation (hypertonia or spasticity), a decrease in tone (hypotonia), or an inappropriate type of activation for the activity in question (eg, rigidity in a person with Parkinson's disease, ataxia with cerebellar disorders).

Adaptation of motor behavior is demonstrated as changes, in muscle activation and motor unit recruitment patterns, that occur in such a way as to minimize the energy expended in meeting a familiar motor goal. Motor learning participates in the adaptation process and can be described as facilitation or streamlining of the middle motor level strategic decision-making process. Performance of a novel motor act may be characterized by any or a combination of the following activation problems:

1. Individual muscle stiffness in excess of that needed to perform the act.
2. Inappropriate slowness in performance of the act.

3. Inappropriate recruitment of sets of muscles as demonstrated by such things as increased co-contraction, increased use of proximal muscles, and increased synergist activation above that seen in the same movement when it is learned.
4. Inappropriate timing of activation of muscles.
5. Production of less than maximally efficient movement trajectories.
6. Errors in termination of movement trajectories.

These problems reflect either a need to maximize sensory input relevant to the performance of the act or the use of minimally efficient decision-making processes. Increased muscle stiffness and slowness of movement increase the availability of proprioceptive information while the act is occurring. This sensory information can then be used in a feedback, corrective mode to adjust motor behavior. In a learned movement, there is minimal need for error detection while the motor act is occurring; the amount of sensory input can be decreased and can be used in a feedforward mode to modify future performances. Errors or inefficiencies in muscle selection and timing of activation can be related to lack of easily available neural pathways controlling selection (gating) and modulation of relevant sensory and system state information. Once a movement has been learned, a single command can elicit the appropriate pattern and sequence of movement components. Before this, individual commands are necessary for each component, and integration is limited among commands. Within the middle level of the hierarchy, the basal ganglia and cerebellum are involved particularly in the aspects of motor learning that set up coordinated patterns of motor commands.

Although specific functions are emphasized in each component of the motor system, all of the hierarchy participates to a greater or lesser extent in the development of all control factors. Under normal circumstances, each component is involved in any movement. Determination of the major function of any component is only possible either under experimental or pathological circumstances in which the component is lost and the function is demonstrable by its absence or when the component is no longer integrated into the system and the function is demonstrated in a released form. Loss of higher levels of the hierarchy may produce either of two possible conditions:

1. Absence of motor activity (even though the lower center is intact) resulting from loss of descending excitatory input.
2. Release of stereotyped motor activity (on the basis of lower center function) resulting from loss of descending inhibitory input.

Given these considerations, a primary goal of any therapy directed at improving sensorimotor function will be the reintegration, to the extent possible, of lower centers into a complete motor control hierarchy.

Types of Motor Behavior

There are four basic classes of motor behavior, each of which uses the whole range of the motor system under normal circumstances. These types in their general order of development are as follows:

1. Movements producing *postural adjustments*.
2. Muscle activation producing *posture maintenance* through co-contraction.
3. *Locomotor* movements.
4. *Fractionated*, goal-directed movements.

More than one type of motor behavior usually is occurring concurrently. The first two types of muscle activation are essential for the production of either locomotor or fractionated behavior.

Movements that produce postural adjustments of the entire body or some part of the body range in complexity from very simply organized sensorimotor reflexes to complex sensorimotor responses. The flexor reflex system, which is organized primarily within the interneurons of the spinal cord, is probably the most simple movement pattern in this class. The other phasic motor responses considered to be in this class of movement include primarily the following:

1. Righting reflexes or responses (eg, body on body, neck righting, labyrinthine righting, optical righting).
2. Equilibrium responses (eg, parachute reaction, propping, hopping).
3. Orienting responses (eg, auditory orienting, visual orienting, placing response of an extremity in response to contact with a surface or object).

Righting reflexes serve to maintain the axial parts of the body in a normal functional relationship to each other or to the external world (Fig. 13-4).

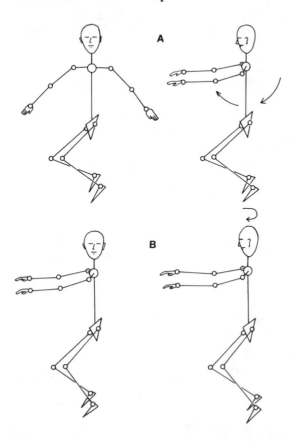

Figure 13-4. Vertebral righting reflexes. A. Body-on-body righting reflex. Rotation of the trunk axis in the lumbar region is followed by rotation of the upper trunk and neck to bring the vertebral column into straight alignment. B. Neck righting on the body. Rotation of the vertebral column in the lower cervical region is followed by upper cervical rotation bringing the head into alignment with the body.

Thus, body righting in response to rotation of one body part on another returns all of the involved parts to a position of straight alignment with each other. Neck righting, triggered by proprioceptors in the neck, brings the head into straight alignment with the upper trunk. Labyrinthine righting, as already discussed in Chapter 9, orients the head upright in relation to gravitational forces. Finally, optical righting moves the eyes and face in such a way as to maintain the face upright and the visual field horizontal (Chap. 16).

Equilibrium responses serve to move the body in such a way as to maintain the center of gravity over the base of support (hopping) or to enlarge the base of support (propping, parachute reaction) (Fig. 13-5). The stimulus is rapid movement of the center of gravity outside of the existing base of support. Orienting responses serve to adjust body and head position in such a way as to bring objects being attended to or used into optimal functional relationship with sensors or the hands or feet (Fig. 13-6). Although righting and equilibrium responses do not require the thalamocortical function of attention for their expression, many orienting responses do. In the case of visual and auditory orienting, there is typically conscious awareness or perception of the orienting stimulus. In placing and orienting behavior of the hand and foot, perception of the stimulus is not always present.

Within each group of postural adjustment movements there is a range of complexity of the neural systems involved and a range of time over which

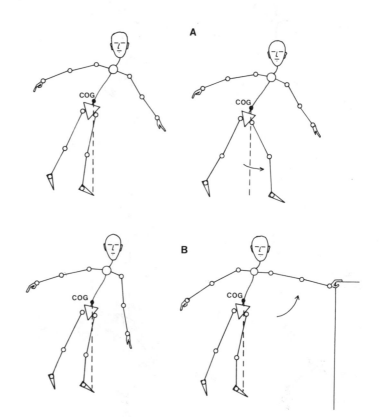

Figure 13-5. Equilibrium responses. A. Hopping response. Disturbance of the upright body so that the center of gravity (COG) is no longer over the base of support is followed by readjustment of the base of support to recenter the center of gravity. B. Propping response. The base of support is broadened in this case by movement of the upper extremity to prop the body against an available support.

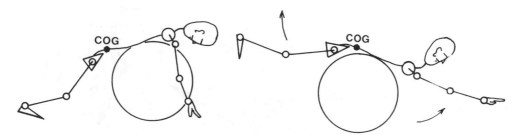

C. Parachute reaction. In the prone position a rapid forward shift of the center of gravity forward over the support leads to extension of all extremities and the vertebral column. The upper extremity extension broadens the base of support while the neck extension assists in head righting.

mature behavior develops. At maturity, all of these behaviors normally use the entire sensorimotor hierarchy in varying degrees. The more complex responses can normally be suppressed voluntarily but are evident when conscious control of the motor system is directed elsewhere.

Posture is maintained not by rigid, static contraction of muscles but by flexible cocontraction of muscles at appropriate joints. In posture maintenance states, muscle stiffness of cocontracting muscle groups is greater than it is during movement states. As a result of this, most of the neural activity related to posture maintenance is concerned with adjusting the ability of alpha motor neurons to respond to changes in muscle length and tension (ie, to maintain constant stiffness). The simplest substrates for postural maintenance activity are found at the spinal level: the Ia and Ib reflex loops. Additional types of activity supporting specific postures include the following:

1. Long loop stretch reflexes through the sensorimotor cortex.
2. Tonic postural reflexes (eg, tonic neck reflexes, tonic labyrinthine reflexes).
3. Cerebellar cocontraction.

Long loop stretch reflexes use the dorsal column proprioceptive projections to area 4 of the cortex. Like the spinal stretch reflex, long loop reflexes respond to a sudden displacement or change in tension (Fig. 13-7). The response occurs in time between the spinal reflex and any voluntary response to the disturbance. Long loop reflexes are variable in sign. Basically, when the disturbance is opposite to the intended movement or tension production, the long loop response is increased activation of the agonist muscle. When the disturbance is in the direction of intended movement, the response is decreased or nonexistent. Long loop reflexes thus illustrate the effect of setting of motor goals on the probability of activation of area 4 pyramidal cells. They have more of a feedforward than a feedback function.

The tonic labyrinthine reflexes have already been described in Chapter 9. Tonic neck reflexes also have a major effect on postural activity in proximal

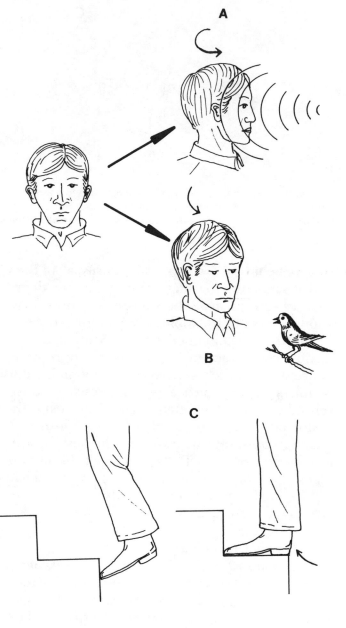

Figure 13-6. Orienting responses. A. Auditory orienting to a sound. The head is turned to equalize the arrival of sound at both ears. B. Visual orienting. The head is turned to center the attended object within both visual fields. C. Placing response in the lower extremity. Tactile contact with the dorsum of the foot leads to readjustment of foot position to permit placement of the sole of the foot on the object. D. Orienting response in the hand. Tactile contact with the hand on any surface other than the radial palmar surface (here, the ulnar palmar surface) leads to readjustment of hand position to permit grasp of the object.

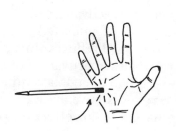

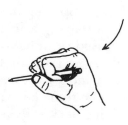

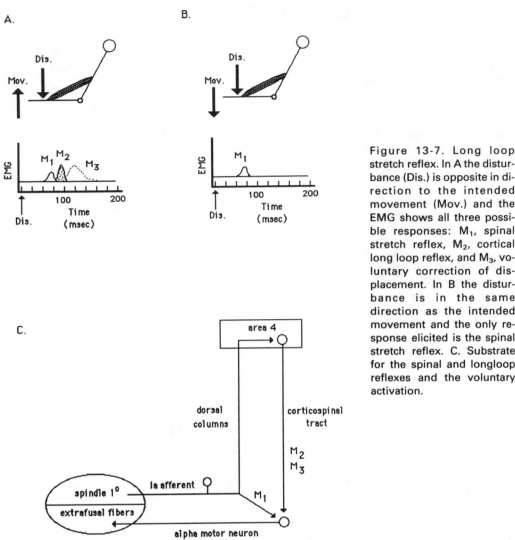

A.

B.

C.

Figure 13-7. Long loop stretch reflex. In A the disturbance (Dis.) is opposite in direction to the intended movement (Mov.) and the EMG shows all three possible responses: M_1, spinal stretch reflex, M_2, cortical long loop reflex, and M_3, voluntary correction of displacement. In B the disturbance is in the same direction as the intended movement and the only response elicited is the spinal stretch reflex. C. Substrate for the spinal and longloop reflexes and the voluntary activation.

limb muscles (Fig. 13-8). When strongly present, they can also effect distal limb muscles. The sensors for the tonic neck reflexes are neck proprioceptors; the integrating center for these reflexes appears to be the interneurons of the cervical region, with descending propriospinal connections. The reticular formation of the brainstem also provides ongoing or tonic control over axial muscles. Generally, the picture demonstrated with release of the descending reticulospinal motor control is one of axial extension. In some cases, extension may also be demonstrated in limb muscles. These circuits are of major importance in modulating the level of excitability of specific alpha motor neurons. Unlike the posture adjustment movements described earlier, it usually is not possible to voluntarily suppress the activity of these postural maintenance

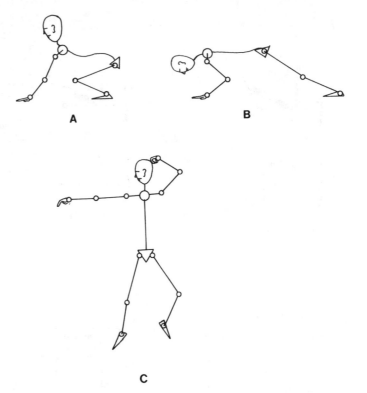

Figure 13-8. Tonic neck reflexes. A and B. Symmetrical tonic neck reflexes. Extension of the neck leads to upper extremity extension, upper trunk extension and lower extremity flexion. Neck flexion results in upper extremity flexion and lower extremity extension. C. Asymmetrical tonic neck reflex. Rotation of the neck leads to upper and lower extremity extension on the side towards which the face is turned and upper and lower extremity flexion on the side away from the face.

activities. This does not indicate a lack of cerebral hemisphere involvement in the production of these activities but rather the overriding importance of control of muscle stiffness for the production of any type of normal motor behavior. When the substrate relevant to production of cocontraction is damaged or is poorly integrated into overall motor control, there is evidence of abnormal tone and of movement decomposition.

Locomotor movements are complex patterns of motor activity that serve the purpose of moving the entire body from one location to another. The movements include behaviors such as leg movements during walking, running, and galloping or other modifications of gait, arm swing, and trunk rotation, all of which normally act concurrently. Locomotor movements are based on relatively simple spinal circuits, among them the flexor-withdrawal, crossed-extension circuit, which automatically produce complementary movements in extremities on the opposite side of the body. There is considerable evidence for a "locomotor center" in the midbrain reticular formation that, at least in lower animals, can operate to produce locomotion in the absence of cortical input. It is likely that in humans control of locomotion has been "corticalized" to a very large extent.

Fractionated, goal-directed movements are those we most typically think of as being "voluntary" (even though many of them are performed, when learned, with virtually no attention being paid to them). Fractionated movement is thought of usually as occurring in distal joints, on the base of proximally stabilized, or cocontracted, joints. However, fractionated movement, or muscle activation, can occur at any joint to a greater or lesser extent, depending on the degree to which control of the necessary alpha motor neurons can be isolated. Fractionated movement, for the sake of efficiency, uses most of the components of motor systems described above; it also requires (at least until learned) conscious activation of sets of specific neurons in area 4 of the sensorimotor cortex.

Classification of Motor Systems

A number of anatomical and functional systems are used for classifying descending motor systems. Because a given anatomical pathway may carry more than one type of functional information, and because a given type of function may be carried out by more than one pathway, correlation between anatomical and functional classification systems is not exact. Two classification systems based primarily on clinical observation are still in common use, even though they really do not adequately describe motor function. One provides a distinction between pyramidal and extrapyramidal systems, with the pyramidal system including motor control projections emanating from the cerebral cortex and the extrapyramidal system including everything else. This classification is functionally quite inaccurate, but it is still somewhat useful clinically in making a very broad distinction between types of motor dysfunction. The second clinical classification system makes a distinction between upper and lower motor neuron dysfunction, with the lower motor neuron referring to alpha motor neurons and the muscle fibers they innervate (the motor unit), and the upper motor neuron referring to any collection of motor control neurons above the level of the spinal cord. Again, this classification system is too general to be of real use in making specific distinctions on the basis of function or even anatomy, but it does retain some clinical usefullness.

Referring back to the classification of types of motor behavior, we could try to establish a corresponding classification of descending motor pathways. Here again there is difficulty due to the evidence that all or most descending pathways are used in varying degrees for the production of any type of motor behavior. However, it is possible to group descending pathways generally into those that primarily function to the adjust and maintain posture and those that primarily produce locomotor and fractionated motor behavior. Such a classification scheme has the advantage of bearing a strong relationship to anatomical distinctions among pathways, in terms of their location within the spinal cord and to a certain extent, in terms of their point of origin in various motor control centers of the nervous system.

In the spinal cord, motor control pathways are grouped anatomically into a dorsolateral system containing the lateral corticospinal and rubrospinal tracts and a ventromedial system containing the vestibulospinal, reticulospinal, anterior corticospinal, and tectospinal tracts and the medial longitudinal fasciculus. The dorsolateral system can be subdivided functionally into a set of fibers that control proximal limb muscles and a set that control distal limb muscles (Fig. 13-9). Proximal control is exerted through both the rubrospinal and the lateral corticospinal pathways; distal control nearly is exclusively the province of the corticospinal tract. Movement of distal joints for the purposes of postural adjustment or maintenance occurs in the foot and ankle during stance. Control of this type of activity very likely involves other pathways besides the lateral corticospinal tract. The importance of the rubrospinal tract for descending motor control in humans is open to some question. The possibility exists that most functions, including locomotion, ascribed to this pathway in quadrupeds and even in other primates have been taken over by corticospinal projections. The lateral corticospinal system is definitely of major importance in the production of fractionated motor behavior, but as stated earlier, it can be used, although with less efficiency, for the production of all other types of motor behavior. The lateral corticospinal and rubrospinal activity is facilitated by lateral reticulospinal pathways from the medulla that act to inhibit spinal postural interneuron activity. The lateral reticulospinal input also acts on the interneurons and gamma motor neurons to facilitate sensory input that will support movement as opposed to maintain posture.

The ventromedial system also can be subdivided into fibers that are engaged primarily in control of axial or trunk muscles and fibers that control proximal limb muscles. Frequently, the control exerted by these systems is somewhat indirect, acting eother through the mechanism of adjusting alpha

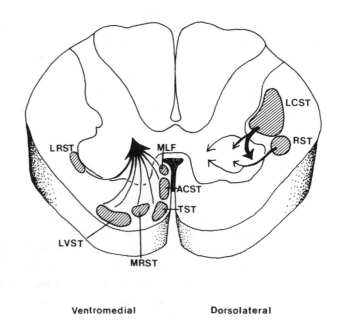

Figure 13-9. Dorsolateral and ventromedial descending somatomotor control systems. The dorsolateral system consists of the lateral corticospinal tract *(LCST)* and the rubrospinal tract *(RST)*. The ventromedial system contains a greater number of pathways, the anterior corticospinal tract *(ACST)*, the lateral reticulospinal tract*(LRST)*, the lateral vestibulospinal tract *(LVST)*, the medial longitudinal fasciculus *(MLF)*, the medial reticulospinal tract *(MRST)*, and the tectospinal tract *(TST)*. The medial longitudinal fasciculus and the tectospinal tract project predominantly to cervical spinal levels. All of these tracts contain sensory modulation as well as the motor control projections illustrated here.

Ventromedial   Dorsolateral

motor neuron excitability through the spinal interneuron system or through tonic synaptic activity. Axial muscles receive control by way of the vestibulospinal, tectospinal (predominantly from the superior colliculus), anterior corticospinal, and medial reticulospinal pathways. Proximal limb muscles receive input primarily from vestibulospinal and lateral reticulospinal pathways. As would be expected, these pathways are most involved in the adjustment and maintenance of posture and are not capable of eliciting fractionated movement. The medial reticulospinal input from the pons provides antigravity posture, with relatively constant excitation to upper limb flexor muscles and lower limb extensors. The effect of the vestibulospinal and tectospinal tracts on alpha motor neuron excitability is variable depending on the sensory information coming into these pathways from their respective sense organs.

It is now recognized that descending motor control pathways convey a great deal of information used for the purpose of modulating sensory and system state activity in various levels of ascending sensory pathways rather than for directing the activity of motor neurons. In some pathways, sensory modulatory fibers considerably outnumber motor control fibers, as is the case in the lateral corticospinal tract. This complex pathway has three major functions:

1. Regulation of activity in lower motor control centers including the red nucleus, the brainstem reticular formation, and the interneurons of the spinal cord.
2. Modulation, or gating, of sensory and system state activity at various levels of the neuraxis.
3. Direction of activity in alpha and gamma motor neurons, either directly or through interneuron systems.

More than half the fibers descending in the lateral corticospinal tract have synapses in the dorsal horn of the spinal cord and in the nuclei of ascending sensory pathways (particularly nucleus gracilis and cuneatus). Fibers that will eventually have synapses in the ventral horn of the spinal cord typically send collateral projections to the red nucleus and the brainstem reticular formation. Cells of origin for the lateral corticospinal tract are located throughout the sensorimotor cortex, with each area differing in the location of its synaptic terminals. Cells that are involved predominantly in sensory modulation arise from areas 3, 1, 2, and possibly 5. Cells in area 6 send information to the ventral horn, probably to bring about changes in motor neuron excitability and very possibly to participate in relatively unfractionated, highly patterned, types of movement. Area 4 projects also to the ventral horn and is most involved in the production of fractionated movement, acting either through spinal interneuronal systems or through monosynaptic contact with alpha (and gamma) motor neurons.

Fractionated movement is produced by the lateral corticospinal pathway through the action of four interdependent behaviors, all of which can be controlled to a very large degree by the pathway acting alone. The first behavior is direct, discrete excitation of specific sets of alpha motor neurons according to patterns established in the sensorimotor cortex. Secondarily, there is related gating of incoming sensory and system state activity by two mechanisms:

1. Enhancement of information related to the desired movement and inhibition of irrelevant information through interaction with ascending pathways in the spinal cord or at higher levels.
2. Enhancement of sensory information appropriate to the specific type of motor activity through regulation of gamma motor neurons.

Finally, the possibility exists of coordinated adjustment of alpha motor neuron excitability through collateral projections to the red nucleus and brainstem reticular formation or through direct interaction with spinal interneuron systems. This last possibility of interaction with spinal interneurons is illustrated particularly by the set of corticospinal fibers that do not decussate in the medulla but descend ipsilaterally in the ventral funiculus of the spinal cord, forming the anterior corticospinal tract.

The size principle that governs recruitment of alpha motor neurons and their motor units also operates in the corticospinal fibers that have synapses directly with alpha motor neurons. Smooth production of tension is controlled by the sequential recruitment of larger motor units (with their larger motor neurons), such that each increment in tension is a relatively small percentage of the existing total tension. In a corresponding fashion, the larger pyramidal cells in area 4 innervate larger alpha motor neurons and are recruited later during motor activities requiring gradual tension development. Smaller pyramidal cells are more important for production of finely graded and precisely controlled motor behavior, particularly in distal extremity joints.

Considerable evidence exists that the activation of pyramidal cells occurs according to probability rather than "all-or-nothing" rules. The frequency of activation of a given pyramidal cell within a set of pyramidal cells that can control a specific movement trajectory can be modulated smoothly, permitting nearly infinite patterns of pyramidal cell activation. The number of possible patterns becomes very limited during the process of motor learning.

The remaining two major components of the middle level (the basal ganglia and the cerebellum) do not send direct descending projections to the spinal cord. As will be discussed in Chapter 14, their major projections are to the limbic and association cortex and the sensorimotor cortex. The effect of their activity thus is projected in large part to the spinal cord through the corticospinal pathway. The cerebellum can additionally affect motor behavior through projections to the vestibular nuclei and reticular formation; the basal ganglia have some projections to the midbrain reticular formation.

To return to the clinical classification systems discussed earlier, the pyramidal system functionally includes the corticospinal projections and all of the brainstem motor centers with which it can interact. Disturbance of the pyramidal system thus is likely to result in alterations of alpha motor neuron excitability (or changes in tone), difficulty in voluntary activation of muscles, and, what is not so often recognized, inappropriate use of sensory information related to movement. Depending on the exact location of a lesion involving this system there may be specific inhibition of certain types of motor behavior or release of various tonic and phasic postural movement patterns. The extrapyramidal system would refer primarily to the basal ganglia and cerebellum which do not have direct spinal projections. Classically, extrapyramidal disorders refer to alterations in motor behavior resulting from the release or loss of motor control generated in the basal ganglia; cerebellar disorders are classed separately. Looking at the upper versus lower motor neuron distinction, lower motor neuron disorders refer to problems arising from the loss of motor units. In such problems, there is no remaining alternate pathway for activation of the involved muscle fibers, which thus are completely paralyzed. Upper motor neuron disorders most typically refer to disorders of the corticospinal pathway, although occasionally disturbances of other higher motor control centers may be included in this classification. Upper motor neuron lesions can theoretically include both pyramidal and extrapyramidal lesions, although the term most often is used for corticospinal tract disorders.

Review Exercises

13-1. One of the many reasons given for using proprioceptive input through guided movements which are normal in appearance (use normal movement trajectories) is that this permits the patient to experience (at either the sensory or the perceptual level or both) the feeling of normal movement. This technique can be effective when the movement is performed with the active assistance of the patient, but is much less effective when the movements are performed passively by the therapist, or are performed against the resistance of hypertonic or inappropriately controlled muscles. Use your understanding of the role of both sensory afferent and control referent (or system state) information during the normal production and learning of movement to support this observation.

13-2. Use palpation and visual observation to determine the differences in specific muscle selection, muscle stiffness, and limb and body posture during performance of first a well-learned (automatic) and then a novel fractionated movement. Observe both the muscles directly involved in producing the movement (agonists and synergists) and more distant muscles which support and position the limb and body. Discuss the advantages, in terms of sensory feedback, to the motor control system of the typical increases in muscle stiffness and decreases in movement speed observed during performance of a novel activity.

The following fractionated movements tend to be novel:
- isolated abduction of the big or little toe
- isolated flexion of a single finger at the middle interphalangeal joint (action of the flexor superficialis)
- reverse supination of the forearm: supination of the proximal end of the ulna and radius at the elbow with external rotation of the humerus while the hand is fixed in pronation

- isolated upper or lower chest breathing, particularly on one side only
- ear wiggling (not possible for many individuals)
- raising one eyebrow (not possible for many individuals)

13-3.   Refer to patient #2 in the Appendix. As you work with this patient you identify a deficiency with isolated, voluntary activation of shoulder abductors on the left side. Suggest three sensory stimulation approaches which could be used to initiate non-fractionated shoulder abduction. Identify approaches which would use each of the following:
   a. a reflex available at the spinal segmental level
   b. a postural adjustment movement
   c. a postural maintenance activity

Discuss:
   1. Could any of the approaches you have suggested be used in combination with each other? If so, how.
   2. If the main intent of obtaining shoulder abduction were to permit normal reaching activity, which of the approaches you have suggested would be most useful? Why?

13-4.   When a vibrator is applied to the tendon of a muscle in such a way that the muscle is repetitively lengthened and shortened with a very small change in actual muscle length there is both a sensory and a motor response. The normal sensory perception is that the muscle is undergoing gradual but consistent lengthening. The reflex motor response is one of increased muscle contraction with either an increase in tension or a decrease in muscle length. Identify and diagram spinal and cortical long loop sensory-motor pathways which could give rise to both the observed perception and the muscle response.

13-5.   Classify the following motor activities as postural adjustments, posture maintenance, locomotor or fractionated movements:
   a. walking
   b. sitting on a stool
   c. kneeling
   d. throwing a ball
   e. writing
   f. catching oneself when falling

13-6.   Refer to Patient #4 in the Appendix.
   a. Describe the types of movements with which you would expect this patient to have difficulty. Would all sets of muscles be affected equally?
   b. As you test for motor function you find that the patient has hyperactive spinal monosynaptic stretch reflexes in the physiological extensor muscles of the left lower extremity. Refer to Figure 13-3 and identify all of the possible reasons why the relevant alpha motor neurons are hyper-responsive to 1a fiber excitation.

13-7. Refer to Patient #2 in the Appendix. If cortical imaging techniques indicate that there is necrosis of most of the cortical and underlying white matter in areas 6, 4, 3, 1, 2 and 5 with relative sparing of the most dorsal parts of these regions, what types of motor function described in this chapter would you expect to be absent or abnormal? What muscles would be affected?

14

Cerebellum and Basal Ganglia

Cerebellar Structure

The cerebellum consists of a midline vermis and two hemispheres. Deep within the hemispheres are three pairs of cerebellar "roof" nuclei. The hemispheres are organized into narrow convolutions, or folia, that have been grouped into a large number of subdivisions. These subdivisions can be grouped either into four functional zones (vestibulocerebellum, vermal zone, intermediate zone, and lateral zone) or into phylogenetic divisions. The two classification systems do not exactly correlate with each other. The roof nuclei consist of a large laterally placed nucleus (dentate nucleus), a doubled intermediate or interpositus nucleus (globose and emboliform), and a medially placed fastigial nucleus.

The cerebellum has three phylogenetic components (Fig. 14-1). The oldest part of the cerebellum, the archicerebellum, is primarily a midline structure. It includes the most anterior and posterior portions of the vermis: the lingula and the nodulus. It also contains two small lateral lobes immediately adjacent to the nodulus: the flocculus. The paleocerebellum includes the remainder of the anterior and posterior portions of the vermis and a small anterior portion of the hemispheres extending posteriorly to the primary fissure. The newest portion of the cerebellum, the neocerebellum, is entirely hemispheric with the exception of a small central vermal component.

Regions of the cerebellum can be classified more functionally in terms of their input-output relationships. Both vermal (lingula and nodulus) and hemispheric (flocculus) portions of the archicerebellum are closely related to the vestibular system (Fig. 14-2). Input is through both vestibular primary afferents and secondary afferents from the vestibular nuclei; output fibers project nearly exclusively to Deiter's (lateral vestibular) nucleus. Thus, the archicerebellum, also called the vestibulocerebellum, has a significant capability for modulating vestibular sensorimotor behavior.

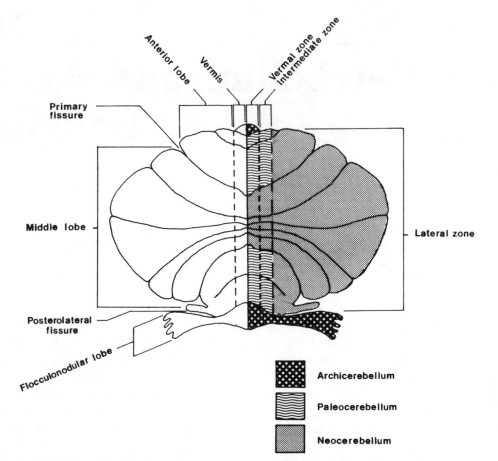

Chapter 14-1. Three classification systems for the cerebellar hemispheres. The cerebellum is viewed from the posterior aspect and flattened. On the left side the major anatomical divisions are outlined. On the right side the major phylogenetic divisions (archicerebellum, paleocerebellum and neocerebellum) are indicated by shading. The major functional zones (vermal, intermediate and lateral) are shown with vertical lines on the right side.

The paleocerebellum is divided into a midline vermal zone and an intermediate zone covering the most medial portions of the hemispheres. Each zone has specific input-output relationships and corresponding functional characteristics. Both zones receive afferent fibers from the spinal cord and trigeminal system (Fig. 14-3). This information is displayed topographically in two head-to-head mirror-image body maps, one in the anterior portion of the cerebellum and one in the posterior portion. Afferent spinal and trigeminal projections to the anterior portion of the cerebellum contain predominantly system state information carried over the ventral (anterior) spinocerebellar tract or its cranial equivalent. Projections to the posterior cerebellum arrive over the dorsal (posterior) spinocerebellar tract and its cranial equivalent and carry proprioceptive and some exteroceptive sensory information. Special sensory information (auditory, vestibular, and visual) is projected into the vermal zone.

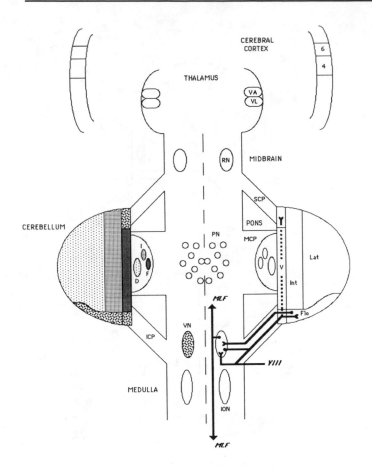

Figure 14-2. Afferent and efferent connections for the vestibulocerebellum. *D*, denate nuc.; *F*, fastigial nuc.; *Flo*, flocculo-nodular lobe; *I*, interpositus nuc.; *ICP*, inferior cerebellar peduncle; *Int*, intermediate zone; *ION*, inferior olivary nucleus; *Lat*, lateral zone; *MCP*, middle cerebellar peduncle; *MLF*, medial longitudinal fasciculus; *PN*, pontine nuclei; *RN*, red nucleus; *SCP*, superior cerebellar peduncle; *V*, vermis; *VA*, ventral anterior nuc. of thalamus; *VL*, ventral lateral nuc. of thalamus; *VN*, vestibular nuclei; *VIII*, VIIIth nerve (vestibular portion).

Efferent fibers from these zones of the cerebellar cortex project to the fastigial nucleus (vermal zone) and the nucleus interpositus (intermediate zone). The fastigial nucleus in turn projects to the spinal cord by way of the vestibular nuclei and the medial longitudinal fasciculus. The nucleus interpositus projects through the superior cerebellar peduncle to the red nucleus. From the red nucleus projections may go to the spinal cord by way of the rubrospinal tract, or to the cerebral hemispheres, predominantly area 6, by way of the ventral anterior and ventral lateral nuclei of the thalamus. The intermediate zone then is connected reciprocally with the motor cortex through corticopontine projections.

The lateral zone of the cerebellum (all neocerebellum) receives input from portions of the sensorimotor cortex by way of the pontine nuclei and some of the pontine reticular formation (corticopontine fibers) (Fig. 14-4). These brainstem nuclei send their fibers by way of the middle cerebral peduncle to the neocerebellum. The output of the lateral zone goes to the dentate nucleus, which in turn projects to the ventral lateral nucleus of the thalamus over the superior cerebellar peduncle and thus to the sensorimotor cortex.

The lateral zone is involved also in a functional loop with the inferior

Figure 14-3. Afferent and efferent connections for the paleocerebellum. A. Connections for the vermis. The primary spinal input arrives over the ventral spinocerebellar tract. The main output to the spinal cord is via the vestibular system and the lateral vestibulospinal tract. B. Connections for the intermediate zone of the cerebellar hemispheres. The spinal input is over the dorsal spinocerebellar tract. Output to the spinal cord is indirect and uses the rubrospinal tract. The intermediate zone also has a connecting loop with the cerebral hemispheres through the red nucleus and the pontine nuclei. *D,* denate nuc.; *DSC,* dorsal spinocerebellar tract; *F,* fastigial nuc.; *Flo,* flocculo-nodular lobe; *I,* interpositus nuc.; *IC,* internal capsule; *ICP,* inferior cerebellar peduncle; *Int,* intermediate zone; *ION,* inferior olivary nucleus; *Lat,* lateral zone; *LVS,* lateral vestibulospinal tract; *MCP,* middle cerebellar peduncle; *PN,* pontine nuclei; *RN,* red nucleus; *RS,* rubospinal tract; *SCP,* superior cerebellar peduncle; *V,* vermis; *VA,* ventral anterior nuc. of thalamus; *VL,* ventral lateral nuc. of thalamus; *VN,* vestibular nuclei; *VSC,* ventral spinocerebellar tract.

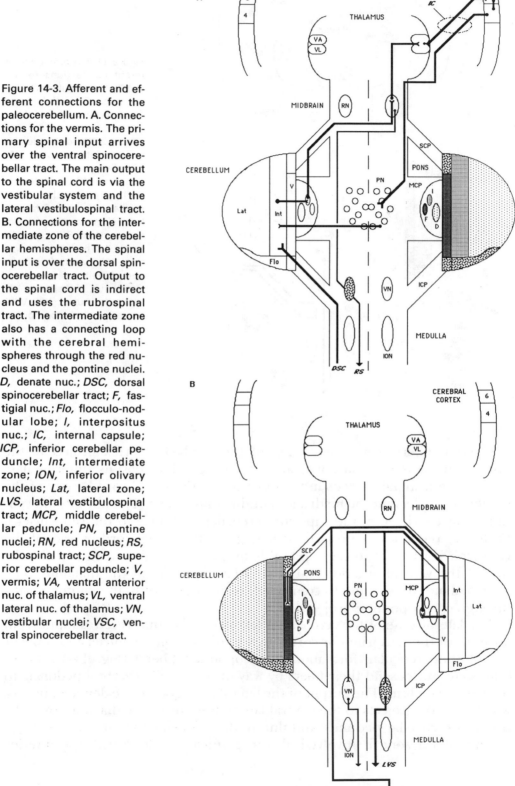

olivary nuclear complex of the medulla (Fig. 14-4). This major medullary nucleus receives proprioceptive and system state information through the spino-olivary tract and collaterals of other ascending pathways, as well as from the vestibular system. It also receives a major input from the red nucleus and collaterals from the corticospinal tract. Its sole output is a crossed projection to the cerebellar hemispheres over the inferior cerebellar peduncle. As a result of the convergence of this varied information dealing with motor behavior, the inferior olivary complex is probably a center for comparing actual with intended motor performance.

Internal Cerebellar Circuitry

The internal circuitry of the cerebellar hemispheres is strikingly simple and uniform. The cerebellar cortex has three cell layers: an external molecular layer with very few cell bodies (basket and stellate cells); a thin, middle Purkinje cell layer; and an internal granular layer with large numbers of Golgi and granule cells (Fig. 14-5). As opposed to the multiple pyramidal cell output pathways in the cerebrum there is only one cerebellar hemisphere output cell: the Purkinje cell. Purkinje cells project to any of the output nuclei of the cerebellum: the roof nuclei and the vestibular nuclei.

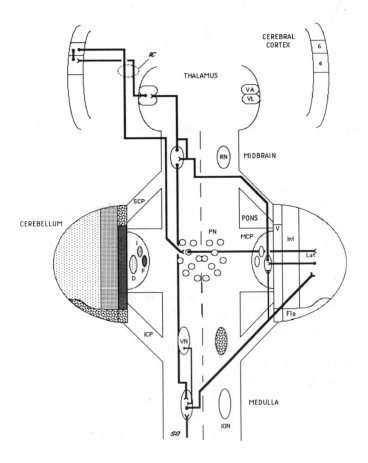

Figure 14-4. Afferent and efferent connections for the neocerebellum (lateral zone). The primary input pathways arise in the inferior olivary nucleus (spinal information and cortical loop) and the pontine nuclei (cortical loop). The output is directed to and through the red nucleus for loops involving the cerebral cortex and the inferior olivary nucleus. *D,* dentate nuc.; *F,* fastigial nuc.; *Flo,* flocculo-nodular lobe; *I,* interpositus nuc.; *IC,* internal capsule; *ICP,* inferior cerebellar peduncle; *Int,* intermediate zone; *ION,* inferior olivary nucleus; *Lat,* lateral zone; *MCP,* middle cerebellar peduncle; *PN,* pontine nuclei; *RN,* red nucleus; *SCP,* superior cerebellar peduncle; *SO,* spino-olivary tract; *V,* vermis; *VA,* ventral anterior nuc. of thalamus; *VL,* ventral lateral nuc. of thalamus; *VN,* vestibular nuclei.

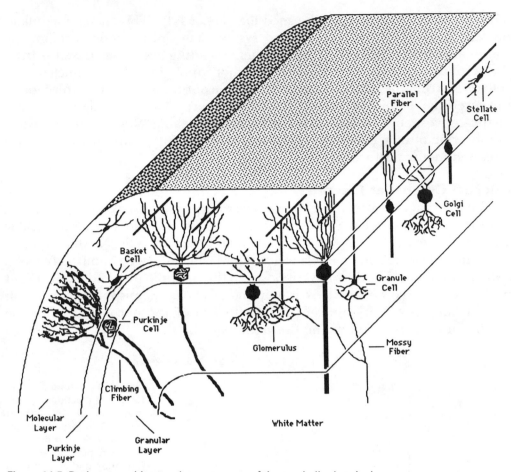

Figure 14-5. Basic cytoarchitectural components of the cerebellar hemispheres.

The internal connections of the cells within the hemispheres are apparently quite stereotyped (Fig. 14-6). Afferent fibers synapsing with Purkinje cells can be classed as either mossy fiber or climbing fiber projections, both of which make excitatory synapses. Mossy fiber projections arise from all the cerebellar afferent pathways already described, with the exception of those from the inferior olive. These afferents communicate with granule cells in the granular layer, which in turn project parallel fibers through the molecular layer. Synapses between mossy fibers and granule cell dendrites are often in the form of complex synaptic glomeruli that also involve the Golgi cells. Each parallel fiber arising from a granule cell communicates with the dendritic fan of about 10 adjacent Purkinje fibers in a single row. Climbing fibers arise from cells in the inferior olivary nuclear complex and form multiple synapses on the main dendritic trunk of a few adjacent Purkinje cells. A given Purkinje cell will receive input from several parallel fibers (mossy fiber system) and from only one climbing fiber. Sets of Purkinje cells receiving convergent climbing and

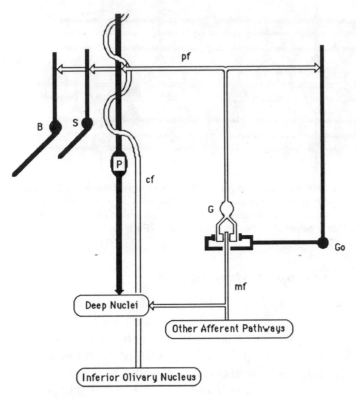

Figure 14-6. Basic pattern of synaptic connections within the cerebellum. The mossy fiber afferents (mf) connect with granule cells (G) in a glomerular structure involving the axons of Golgi cells (Go). Mossy fibers also send collateral projections to corresponding cerebellar deep nuclei. The continuation of this afferent system, the parallel fiber (pf), synapses with the dendritic fan of the Purkinje cell (P) as well as with dendrites of basket (B), stellate (S) and Golgi cells. The climbing fiber (cf) afferents from the inferior olivary nucleus make extensive synaptic contact with Purkinje cell dendritic fans. The Purkinje cell provides the only output from the cerebellar cortex. Due to the extensive number of inhibitory cell types there is a predominance of inhibitory modeling of neural activity within the cerebellar cortex.

mossy fiber projections form microzones in the cerebellar hemispheres (Fig. 14-7). Microzones are the functional units of the cerebellar cortex, analogous to barrels in the cerebral hemispheres. Negative feedback and surround inhibition helping to define microzones is provided by the stellate and basket cells acting on the Purkinje cells and by the Golgi cells acting on the granule cells.

Mossy fiber input to the Purkinje cells elicits tonic activity in the form of chains of simple spikes, or action potentials. Climbing fiber input causes a prolonged depolarization of the Purkinje cells that facilitates simple spike generation, leading to the formation of complex spikes. At the level of the cerebellar nuclei, the simple tonic activity caused by mossy fiber input is periodically inhibited strongly by complex spike activity from the Purkinje cells. The climbing fiber projection to the cerebellum thus may be the means of enabling the cerebellum to inform the cerebral cortex concerning needed adaptive changes in ongoing or anticipated motor programs. The Purkinje cell inhibitory modulation of cerebellar output has been implicated as the basis for certain aspects of adaptation, learning, and memory, related to motor function.

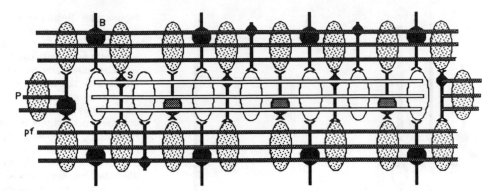

Figure 14-7. Synaptic development of cerebellar cortical microzones. A group of parallel fibers (pf, white) excites a number of Purkinje cells (P, white). They also excite stellate cells (S) in the same region, which in turn inhibit adjacent parallel sets of Purkinje cells. Basket cells (B) also assist in producing effective surround inhibition. The result is selective activation of a group of Purkinje cells.

Basal Ganglia Structure

The basal ganglia are a set of nuclei located deep in the cerebral hemispheres, the diencephalon, and the midbrain. They function as side, or parallel processing, loops for both the motor and homeostatic control systems. At this time, the discussion will be concerned primarily with those portions of the basal ganglia and their interconnecting circuitry that are involved directly in modulating motor behavior. Anatomic classification of the basal ganglia is outlined in Figure 14-8.

The basal ganglia may be viewed as an interrupted cell column extending from the midbrain to the cerebral hemispheres, in close association with the efferent fibers from the hemispheres, namely the corticospinal, corticobulbar, and corticopontine projections (Fig. 14-9). In the midbrain and diencephalon (subthalamus), the basal ganglia lie dorsomedial to these projections that form the cerebral peduncles. In transit between the diencephalon and the cerebral hemispheres, the hemispheric projections (internal capsule) transect the basal ganglia cell column so that the lenticular nuclei now lie lateral and ventral to them. The remaining part of the striatum, the caudate nucleus, still lies dorsomedial to the hemispheric fibers but is connected anteriorly with the putamen. The caudate is an example of a number of structures located in the dorsal diencephalon and cerebral hemispheres in close relationship to the lateral ventricles. During development, the caudate enlarges along with the ventricles to stretch out into a C-curved structure making contact with the ventricles over most of their extent.

There are four clearly identified functional loops through the basal ganglia by which motor information is processed. The basic pathway is similar in all cases and involves entry into the basal ganglia at one of the main entry nuclei (caudate, putamen, subthalamic nucleus, nucleus accumbens), transfer to "internal" basal ganglia nuclei (globus pallidus external, substantia nigra pars compacta), and release to the thalamus or brainstem by way of an exit nucleus

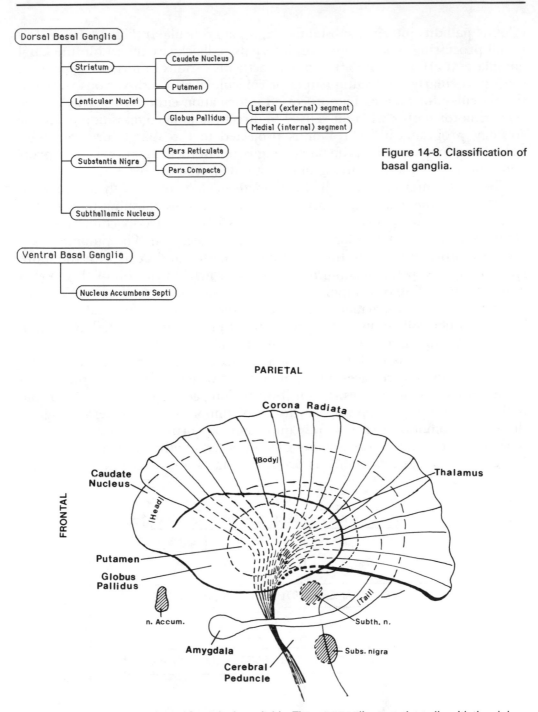

Figure 14-8. Classification of basal ganglia.

Figure 14-9. Basal ganglia viewed from the lateral side. The putamen lies most laterally with the globus pallidus immediately medial to it. The globus pallidus is separated from the thalamus by the posterior limb of the internal capsule. The anterior limb of the internal capsule separates the body and part of the head of the caudate from the putamen. The subthalamic nucleus and the substantia nigra are medial and dorsal to the cortical projecting fibers in the cerebral peduncles. The amygdala lies in the anterior tip of the temporal lobe immediately adjacent, but not actually connected, to the tail of the caudate. The nucleus accumbens lies within the septal region of the frontal lobe.

(globus pallidus internal, substantia nigra pars reticulata) (Fig. 14-10). Additional processing typically involves internal feedback circuits within the basal ganglia and afferent and efferent contact with various brainstem structures, most particularly the tectum (superior colliculus), and with various nuclei in the reticular formation. The processed information either is returned to the sensorimotor cortex where it is used to direct the final composition of motor strategy programs in area 4 or is projected to the spinal cord. Separate processing loops through the basal ganglia retain their identity, with convergence of information occurring only as it is delivered to area 4.

The loop entering through the caudate nucleus deals with information generated in the association cortex and involved in establishing motor goals and general motor plans. By means of processing in this loop, components of complex motor behaviors may be selected and integrated. The putamen loop receives information from the sensorimotor cortex and deals with the more specific aspects of formulating motor plans. A major function of this loop is appropriate scaling of components of complex movements. The subthalamic nucleus receives information from area 4, either from corticospinal and corticobulbar fiber collaterals or by way of direct projections. It thus can serve a comparator function between actual and intended motor commands. Each of these loops projects back to the motor cortex by way of the thalamus. The nucleus accumbens receives information from various portions of the association cortex and integrates it with information received generally from the limbic system. This loop appears to be of importance in generating goal-directed locomotion that may rely minimally on cortical motor area activity. To what extent this is true in humans as opposed to other animals is unclear; however the nucleus accumbens probably retains a central role in enabling

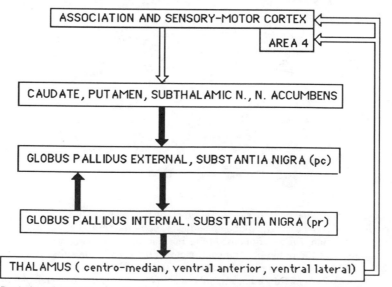

Figure 14-10. Basic basal ganglia—cortical loops through the thalamus.

locomotor behavior. A major projection of this loop is to the midbrain reticular formation. In quadrupeds, the midbrain reticular formation has an important role in the generation of locomotor activity.

Each set of basal ganglia receives both ipsilateral and contralateral cortical projections. This duality of cortical input does not necessarily provide a safety factor if one side of the basal ganglia ceases to operate. The duality more likely provides for integration of motor information that is generated in both sides of the cortex but that is to be expressed by one or the other side of the body. This integration enables bilateral coordination of motor behavior and reinforces the interhemispheric communication provided by the corpus callosum.

Cerebellar and Basal Ganglia Function

Parallel processing of motor plans through the cerebellar and basal ganglia side loops acts essentially to enable and trigger motor behavior that is efficient and functionally integrated with all other current activity in the body. Together, these loops permit a high degree of automaticity in even complex motor behaviors, such as locomotion. The automaticity frees cortical attention circuits involved in conscious processing for other tasks than can then occur concurrently with motor behavior. The value of this can be estimated if you try performing a relatively simple intellectual task, such as adding numbers, while at the same time attempting an unfamiliar motor act.

The cerebellum is involved in triggering specific motor commands. Output from the cerebellum is of greatest importance in determining appropriate timing and intensity of motor unit activation. The vermal and intermediate zones, by virtue of their sensory and system state afferents, are involved in regulating motor unit activity through integration, or comparison, of cortical commands (efference copies of intended movement) and information concerning actual behavior (reference copies of actual movement). These zones are of importance in directing ongoing motor activity such as might be seen in postural maintenance or cocontraction. The lateral zone instructs the motor cortex concerning "starts" and "stops" of motor patterns or their components. This information is essential for the efficient performance of motor behavior that does not permit ongoing error correction (open loop behavior) such as goal-directed ballistic movements, locomotion, and possibly postural adjustment movements. The comparator abilities of the inferior olivary nuclear complex are involved in the adjustments of motor commands initiated by the cerebellum. Complex spike activity resulting from climbing fiber activation of Purkinje cells has a timing that makes it appropriate as a substrate for adapting and learning motor patterns.

The four loops through the basal ganglia already described provide "enabling" input to the motor system. Enabling input is basically excitatory, although it almost certainly involves surround inhibition. The input makes the target cells particularly receptive to specific additional excitatory input, although it does not itself directly elicit activity in the target cells. (It can be thought of as being analogous to the permissive behavior of certain hormones.) Enabling activity in the basal ganglia is probably both intrinsic and extrinsic in nature. Within the basal ganglia, constant activity in certain nuclei, particularly the substantia nigra and globus pallidus and possibly the striatum, is probably essential for appropriate processing of commands entering the striatum and subthalamic nucleus. The constant, or tonic, internal activity is cycled among the various nuclei of the basal ganglia through the internal feedback loops. Tonic input from the brainstem, which can vary with the degree of arousal and possibly the type of incoming sensory information available, is used also in supporting and modifying motor control processing in the basal ganglia. The output from the basal ganglia to the various cortical motor regions (or, in the case of the nucleus accumbens, to the midbrain locomotor center) also is enabling in nature. Within the basal ganglia selection and promotion of specific components and qualities of movement apparently involves "inhibitory sculpting" through surround inhibition. This inhibitory sculpting depends on the presence of tonic excitation in a circuit and brings about enhancement of the differences between pathways that are specifically activated and those that are uninvolved in a particular event.

Patterns of Dysfunction of the Cerebellum and Basal Ganglia

The normal functions of the basal ganglia and the cerebellum have been deduced not only from a variety of experimental studies but also from careful observation of clinical states that can be attributed to dysfunction involving these parts of the motor system.

Cerebellar system dysfunction leads to inability either to adjust ongoing movements correctly in response to changes in the environment or to initiate or stop muscle activity at appropriate times. These difficulties may be expressed as ataxia, in which timing of generation of muscle tension is not coordinated; generalized tone abnormalities (frequently hypotonia); and *intention* tremor, which occurs during movement. Although basal ganglia disorders are associated most typically with pathology localized to the basal ganglia themselves, cerebellar disorders may result from pathology either within the cerebellum or in its numerous afferent and efferent pathways. In many cases, cerebellar disorders are not as localized to specific body parts as basal ganglia disorders, suggesting a large amount of somatotopically convergent or overlapping processing in this system.

Basal ganglia disorders may produce various dyskinesias, bradykinesis, or tremor, alone or in combination. Dyskinesias are abnormal movement patterns characterized by inappropriate scaling and integration of components of complex motor behaviors. They include the general types listed below:

1. Chorea: jerky, dance-like movements of the extremities or neck.

2. Ballismus: abrupt throwing or twisting movements of the extremities, trunk, or neck.
3. Athetosis: slow, sustained abnormal postural adjustment movements of the extremities or neck.
4. Tardive or facial dyskinesia: involuntary movements of muscles innervated by cranial nerves VII, XII, and V.

The observation that these dyskinesias and other basal ganglia disorders may be quite localized supports the hypothesis that motor control processing in the basal ganglia is segregated rather strictly by body regions rather than being global.

The various components of the basal ganglia control different qualities of movement. As a result, damage of discrete portions of the basal ganglia leads to different types of movement disorder (Fig. 14-11). Bradykinesis and tremor are likely the result of alteration in the ongoing tonic activity of the internal feedback circuits of the basal ganglia. In bradykinesis, there is a diminished amount and flexibility of movement and an inability to adjust scaling of movement, resulting in stereotyped behavior of limited range. Bradykinesis also is associated typically with rigidity, a state in which there is abnormal cocontraction during goal-directed and postural adjustment movements and locomotion. The tremor seen with basal ganglia disorders is a *resting* tremor, evident only when no movement is intended. It may be due to release from tonic inhibition of pace-maker type activity in the striatum.

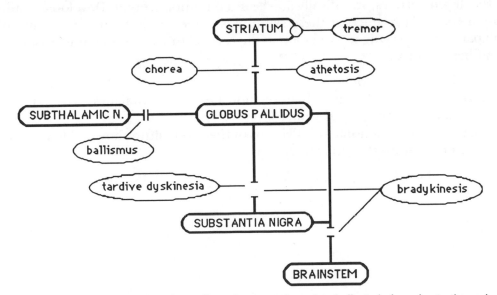

Figure 14-11. Interruption of basal ganglia pathways at the points indicated gives rise to the various types of pathology shown.

Review Exercises

14-1.   Develop a circuit diagram for the putamen loop of the basal ganglia which incorporates parallel pathways, surround inhibition and pacemaker activity. Arrange the pathway in such a way that it could be used to 1) selectively enable cells in area 4 which excite elbow flexor motor neurons and 2) selectively inhibit cells in area 4 which excite elbow extensor motor neurons.

14-2.   A person with athetosis exhibits slow but fairly continuous movements of the extremities. This characteristic motor behavior may be interrupted by sudden movements which can resemble postural adjustment movements. The overall posture may present an extreme of postural maintenance patterns in axial muscles. Given this information, refer to Figure 14-11 and describe what type of basal ganglia activity may be released from normal cortical control in persons with athetosis.

14-3.   Refer to Figures 14-6 and 14-7. Develop a network diagram which explains how a proprioceptor could send an error signal to the cerebellum which would result in the transmission of an excitatory corrective signal from the dentate nucleus to the cerebral cortex. Include all relevant cerebellar cells in your diagram, particularly cortical and roof nuclei output cells.

14-4.   Multiple sclerosis is a disease in which myelin in the central nervous system is destroyed in a relatively random fashion. Some of the motor symptoms of multiple sclerosis are those which one would expect to see with cerebellar disorders, specifically ataxia and intention tremor. Develop a justification for the presence of these symptoms based on your understanding of the pathways carrying information to the cerebellum and the characteristics of the fibers involved.

14-5.   Structural Models
   a. Basal ganglia showing their relationship to the thalamus, the internal capsule and the lateral ventricles
   b. Any of the functional subdivisions of the cerebellum showing their major afferent and efferent connections

15

Substrate for Homeostasis

Homeostasis involves integration of behavior among various organs and systems. Regulation of homeostasis occurs through the combined activity of the autonomic component of the nervous system and the endocrine system. The general control system for homeostatic behavior can be described in a way as a hierarchy similar to that used to describe somatomotor control (Fig. 15-1). The higher level of control has the limbic system and the association cortex as its substrate. (Refer to Chap. 18 for a description of the limbic system). This higher level is involved in the type of goal setting that determines the homeostatic needs of the person and the priority for meeting specific needs. The middle level, which is involved in determining the strategies to be used in meeting goals or homeostatic needs, includes primarily the hypothalamus and certain less well-understood parts of the basal ganglia and cerebellum. The lower level, as in the somatomotor system, is divided into several sublevels. Within the nervous system, these are 1) the brainstem reticular formation with associated cranial nerve nuclei, 2) the spinal cord, and 3) the peripheral components of the autonomic nervous system and the myenteric nervous system. Outside the nervous system, the lower level components are the pituitary (all components) and the other endocrine glands. There are several obvious substrate differences between the components of the somatomotor control hierarchy and the homeostatic system. Primary among these are the following:

1. Inclusion of hormonal control substrate and neural substrate.
2. Addition of a relatively independent peripheral neural system.
3. Dual control (excitatory and inhibitory) of effector organs and of central neurons.

Significant functional differences also exist between the somatomotor hierarchy and the homeostatic one. Generally, the homeostatic system is characterized by increased functional autonomy of components of the lower and middle levels of the hierarchy; greater availability of tonic behaviors; and minimization of cortical, voluntary control for either goal setting or strategic planning.

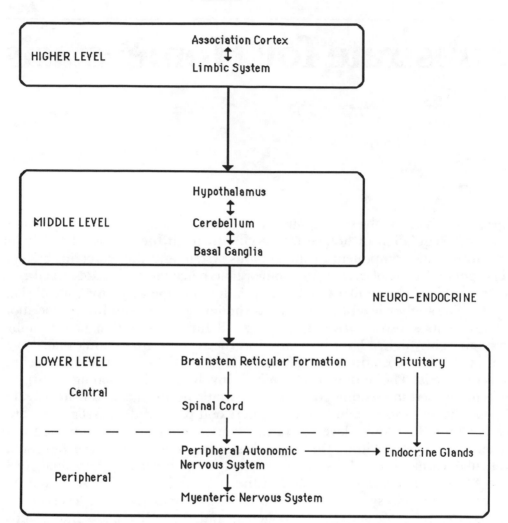

Figure 15-1. Hierarchy of substrate in the homeostatic control system. Neural and neuro-endocrine systems work in parallel.

Activity in the homeostatic control system is dependent on sensory and system state information in much the same way as the somatomotor system (Fig. 15-2). Sensory information is provided by two general groups of receptors sensitive to changes in homeostatic state: peripheral receptors and receptors located within the CNS. System state information is provided both through pathways within the CNS that permit lower level components to report their state of activity to higher levels and through hormonal feedback systems either operating completely in the periphery or interacting with the pituitary and hypothalamus. Information held in memory also is used typically as a basis for determining homeostatic behavior.

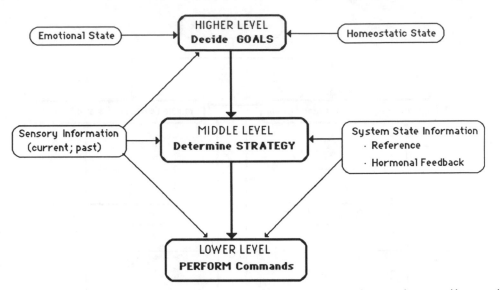

Figure 15-2. Sensory and system-state information input to the homeostatic control system. Hormonal feedback systems play an important role in providing system state information.

The above discussion indicates that the somatomotor and homeostatic systems can be viewed as both structurally and functionally parallel in many ways. This should not be taken to mean that the two control systems operate separately. On the contrary, homeostatic and somatomotor behaviors are closely interactive and typically mutually supportive (Fig. 15-3). Links between the two systems are found at a number of levels:

1. Sensory information related to either skeletal motor or homeostatic activity is projected at many levels to both systems.
2. General information in memory is available to both systems although specific operating memory may be limited to one or the other system.
3. Both systems use the association cortex as a common location for information processing to establish goals.
4. Motor commands generated in either system are transmitted through collateral pathways to the control centers in the other system.

Autonomic Nervous System

Neural substrate that can be considered to be exclusively part of the autonomic nervous system include the following:

1. Postganglionic neurons.
2. Peripheral ganglia and plexi.
3. Preganglionic neurons with their cell bodies either in the intermediolateral horn of the spinal cord or in the general visceral efferent cranial nerve nuclei.

The myenteric plexus of the gut also can be considered as part of the autonomic nervous system, although both in structure and in function it has

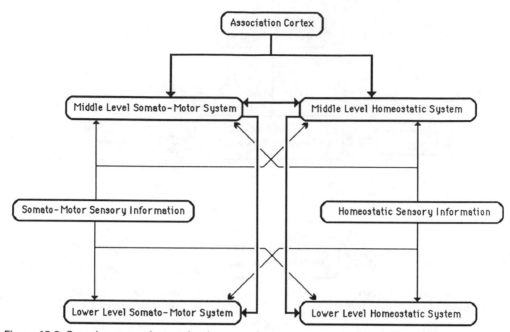

Figure 15-3. Complementary interaction between the somatomotor and homeostatic control systems. Information sharing relies on the use of both divergence of sensory information to separate control centers and convergence of separate sensory information on shared control centers.

considerable independence from the postganglionic fibers which synapse with it. Within the CNS the tracts or neurons connecting the brainstem reticular formation and the preganglionic cell bodies in the spinal cord or brainstem may have exclusively autonomic function, but they may also, through collaterals, influence other aspects of central neural function. The same is true of tracts or neurons from visceral afferent nuclei bringing homeostatic sensory information to the brainstem reticular formation.

Both sensory and motor autonomic innervation of the periphery is organized in a generally somatotopic fashion, but less precisely than is true for the somatic system. The structural organization of the sympathetic peripheral ganglia, as illustrated earlier in Chapter 2 (Fig. 2-11), permits either somatotopically specific innervation of peripheral organs or more diffuse innervation. Parasympathetic innervation appears grossly to be diffuse, but at the individual neuron level it can be somatotopically specific. The dual control of the periphery mentioned earlier is provided typically by the sympathetic system originating in the thoracic and upper lumbar spinal cord (T1-L3), and by the parasympathetic system originating in the general visceral efferent nuclei of the brainstem and preganglionic neurons in the sacral spinal cord (Fig. 15-4). Structural dual innervation permits flexibility in peripheral control of end organs. Classically, the sympathetic and parasympathetic controls were conceived as being both antagonistic to each other and global in effect (ie, all-or-nothing activation of entire systems and thus global response behaviors such as "fight or flight"). A more appropriate concept would be that of the two

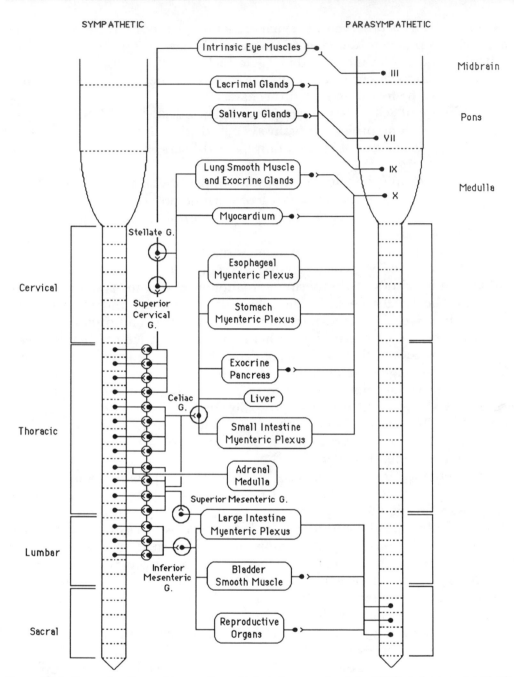

Figure 15-4. General pattern of innervation of internal organs by sympathetic and parasympathetic motor fibers. Vascular smooth muscle and skin sweat and piloerector innervation has been omitted for clarity; the innervation is uniquely sympathetic and arises from all levels of the thoracic and lumbar cord.

systems providing graded modulation of ongoing behavior in the end organs, coupled with integration of internal organ behavior throughout the body. Such a concept permits inclusion of mutually supportive activities of the two systems, such as is observed in sexual responses, without having to consider these as exceptions to the rule of autonomic behavior. The functional dual control of end organs is outlined in Table 15-1.

Relative independence of peripheral control in the autonomic system is supported by the following structural characteristics:

1. Presence of cell bodies in ganglia and plexi outside the CNS.
2. Relatively long projection pathways outside the CNS.
3. The exclusive use of small, unmyelinated fibers as axons for postganglionic neurons.
4. Variability in specificity of synapses with peripheral end organs.
5. Availability of peripheral reflex loops that do not involve the CNS.
6. Divergent projections of preganglionic neurons from any given spinal level or cranial nerve.
7. Availability of coinnervation of end organs.
8. Multiplicity of types of receptors in end organs.

These characteristics of the peripheral autonomic nervous system correlate well with the functional differences between autonomic and somatomotor systems. Relatively slow and persistent modification of end-organ activity is supported by the presence of peripheral synapses, the length of peripheral projection pathways, the use of small diameter postganglionic neurons, and the diffuse arrangement of some nerve-effector synapses. This anatomical arrangement should not be taken to mean that *all* autonomic activity must occur slowly; some can occur very rapidly. In addition, patterns of control within the CNS are of significantly greater importance in determining the speed and persistence of autonomic activation than are the nature of the peripheral anatomical substrate.

The potential for independent function of peripheral components is strongly related to the availability of reflex loops involving neurons that are completely outside the CNS. Relatively extensive reflex activation can occur without viable central connections. In some cases, as discussed earlier when considering pain mechanisms, sensory neurons located in the autonomic nerves appear able to transmit information both orthodromically and antidromically. Activation of such neurons can lead to release of transmitter substances in the periphery as well as at normal synapses. Peripheral independence is enhanced also by the ability of most, if not all, of the end organs innervated by the autonomic nervous system to modulate their activity in the complete absence of neural control.

Stereotyped behavior directed by the autonomic nervous system is supported by divergent projections from individual cranial and spinal nerves. This arrangement can permit single control centers in the CNS to modulate activity efficiently in a large number of end organs. This type of behavior retains generally similar characteristics with each occurrence, but it can be tuned finely to meet the specific requirements of any given event. It can be compared to a certain extent with somatomotor postural adjustment and maintenance activity, which also is stereotyped to a very large extent.

TABLE 15-1. Responses of End Organs to Sympathetic and Parasympathetic Activity

End Organ	Adrenergic Receptor	Response to Adrenergic Input	Response to Cholinergic Input
INTRINSIC EYE MUSCLES			
Radial Muscle, Iris	alpha	contraction	none
Sphincter Muscle, Iris		none	contraction
Ciliary Muscle	beta	relaxation	contraction
LACRIMAL GLANDS		none	increased activity
HEART			
S-A Node	beta-1	increased rate	decreased rate
Atria	beta-1	· increased contractility · increased cond. vel.	decreased contractility decreased cond. vel.
A-V Node	beta-1	increased cond. vel.	decreased cond. vel.
Ventricular Cond. Fibers	beta-1	increased cond. vel.	decreased cond. vel.
Ventricle	beta-1	· increased contractility · increased automaticity	decreased contractility
VASCULAR SMOOTH MUSCLE			
	alpha	contraction	dilation (? humans)
	beta-2	relaxation	
LUNG			
Bronchial Muscle	beta-2	relaxation	contraction
Bronchial Glands	beta-2	decreased activity	increased activity
G-I SYSTEM			
Sphincter Muscles	alpha	contraction	relaxation
Other G-I Muscles	beta-2	relaxation	contraction
Glands	alpha	decreased activity	increased activity
Gallbladder	alpha	relaxation	contraction
SALIVARY GLANDS	alpha	K^+, H_2O secretion	K^+, H_2O secretion
	beta	amylase secretion	
SPLEEN	alpha, beta	contraction or relaxation	none
LIVER	beta-2	glycogenolysis gluconeogenesis	glycogen synthesis
PANCREAS			
Acini	alpha	decreased activity	increased activity
Beta Cells	alpha	decreased activity	increased activity
ADIPOCYTES	beta-2	lipolysis	none
URINARY BLADDER			
Detrusor Muscle	beta-2	relaxation	contraction
Trigone and Sphincter	alpha	contraction	relaxation
UTERUS	alpha, beta	pregnant: contraction nonpregnant: relaxation	variable
PENIS	alpha, beta	ejaculation	erection
SKIN			
Piloerector muscles	alpha	contraction	none
Sweat glands			
· emotional sweating	alpha	increased activity	none
· thermal sweating		none	increased activity
ADRENAL MEDULLA		none	secretion of catecholamines
PINEAL GLAND	beta-2	melatonin secretion	none

Hypothalamic and Pituitary Anatomy

The hypothalamus is the most ventral and anterior portion of the diencephalon, forming a narrow layer of nuclei and associated tracts on either side of the third ventricle immediately below the dorsal thalamus and anterior and medial to the subthalamus. It contains the only portion of the diencephalon clearly visible in a ventral view of the whole brain: the mammillary bodies. The dorsal and ventral boundaries of the hypothalamus are clear: dorsally the hypothalamic sulcus separates the hypothalamus from the thalamus, and ventrally the hypothalamus is either adjacent to the ventral subarachnoid space or continuous with the stalk of the pituitary. The most anterior nucleus of the hypothalamus, the preoptic nucleus, lies immediately below the anterior commissure and dorsal to the optic chiasm. Posterior and lateral regions of the hypothalamus blend into adjacent regions of the temporal lobe, subthalamus, and midbrain.

Hypothalamic nuclei are, understandably, very small and do not always have clearly defined boundaries. The lateral hypothalamic area is broken up extensively with fibers of passage belonging to the medial forebrain bundle. The periventricular area immediately adjacent to the third ventricle is a thin sheet of cells with minimal nuclear organization. The medial region, separated from the lateral region by the fibers of the fornix, contains relatively well-defined nuclei (Fig. 15-5). Functional classification of hypothalamic nuclei

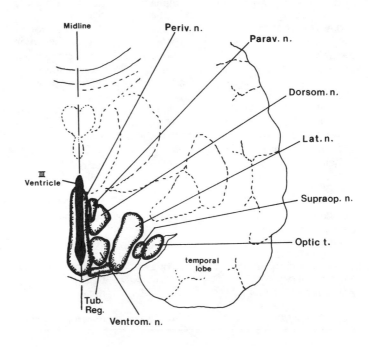

Figure 15-5. Hypothalamic nuclei. A. Coronal section through the hypothalamus.

A

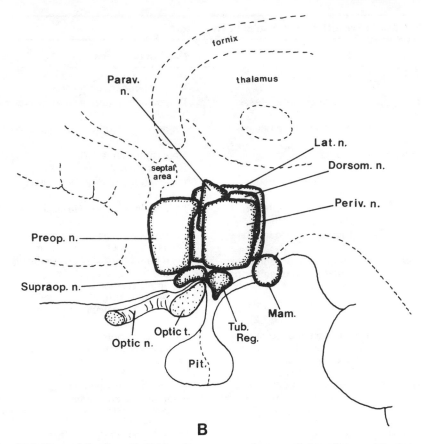

B

B. Midsagittal view of the hypothalamus. *Dorsom. n.,* dorsomedial nuclear region; *Lat. n.,* lateral nuclear region; *Mam.,* mammillary body; *Parav. n.,* paraventricular nucleus; *Periv. n.,* periventricular nuclear region; *Pit.,* pituitary; *Preop. n.,* preoptic nucleus; *Supraop. n.,* supraoptic nucleus; *Tub. Reg.,* tuberal region; *Ventrom. n.* ventromedial nuclear region.

bears little or no relationship to the anatomic organization of the hypothalamus. Those hypothalamic nuclei with clear relationships to the functions to be discussed in the next chapter are described in Table 15-2.

The hypothalamus is linked closely with the limbic system and frontal association cortex through several major pathways including the fornix, stria terminalis, medial forebrain bundle with its continuing cingulate tract, and the mammillothalamic tract (Fig. 15-6 and Table 15-3). The fornix and stria terminalis will be described in more detail with the remainder of the limbic system. The medial forebrain bundle connects the hypothalamus rostrally with the septal region of the frontal lobes and continues on as the cingulate tract with connections to the cingulum and the frontal association cortex. The mammillothalamic tract connects the mammillary nuclear complex to the anterior nucleus of the thalamus, which in turn projects to the cingulum and the frontal association cortex.

Major pathways connecting the hypothalamus to the brainstem include the

TABLE 15-2. Major Hypothalamic Nuclei or Regions

Nucleus	Function	Major Connections
Preoptic	thermoregulation	To: lateral posterior region, hypothalamus To: anterior n. hypothalamus
Supraoptic	neurohormone release	To: posterior pituitary via hypothalamo-hypophyseal tract
Paraventricular	neurohormone release	To: posterior pituitary via hypothalamo-hypophyseal tract
Suprachiasmatic	diurnal cycling	From: optic nerve To: pineal body
Periventricular	regulation of anterior pituitary system	To: anterior pituitary via pituitary portal
Tuberal	regulation of anterior pituitary system	To: anterior pituitary via pituitary portal
Lateral	regulation of food intake	To: septal area via medial forebrain bundle To: limbic system via cingulum
Ventromedial	· regulation of food intake · integration of emotional states and homeostatic activity	From: limbic system (amygdala) via stria terminalis To: limbic system To: reticular formation via dorsal longitudinal fasciculus and central tegmental tract
Dorsomedial	integration of emotional states and homeostatic activity	To: limbic system To: reticular formation via dorsal longitudinal fasciculus and central tegmental tract
Mammillary	integration of emotional states and homeostatic activity	To: anterior n. thalamus via mammillothalamic tract To: periaqueductal grey via mammillo-tegmental tract From: hippocampus via fornix

medial forebrain bundle, the mammillotegmental tract, and the central tegmental tract (Fig. 15-6). Through these bidirectional pathways there is communication between the hypothalamus and various portions of the brainstem reticular formation. The medial forebrain bundle also serves as an internal pathway within the hypothalamus.

The pathways indicated above connect the hypothalamus with other neural regions in the homeostatic control hierarchy. Additionally, there are pathways connecting the hypothalamus with the pituitary. The supraoptic and paraventricular nuclei project into the posterior pituitary through the neurohypophyseal tract. The axon terminals of these fibers release their neurohormones directly into the general circulation rather than into a neural synapse. In a similar fashion, a number of hypothalamic nuclei, primarily medially and ventrally placed, release their neurohormones into the pituitary portal system by which they are transported to the anterior pituitary. In this location the neurohormones act as either releasing or inhibiting factors controlling pituitary hormone release. The major hypothalamic tracts are summarized in Table 15-3.

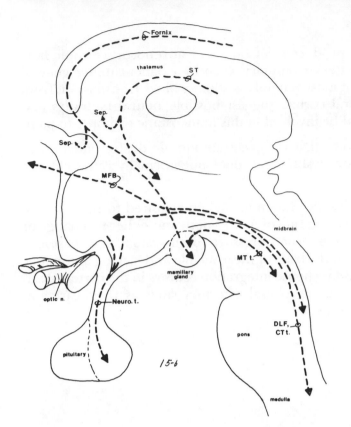

Figure 15-6. Major afferent and efferent hypothalamic pathways. Hypothalamic-brainstem connections include the dorsolateral fasciculus *(DLF)*, the central tegmental tract *(CTt)* and the mammillotegmental tract *(MTt)*. The medial forebrain bundle *(MFB)* connects the brainstem, hypothalamus and ventral regions of the frontal lobes. The neurohypophyseal tract *(Neuro. t)* projects from the hypothalamus to the posterior pituitary. Major afferent limbic tracts to the hypothalamus include the fornix and the stria terminalis *(ST)*, both of which also project to the septal region *(Sep.)*.

TABLE 15-3. Major Afferent and Efferent Pathways for the Hypothalamus

Pathway	Origin	Termination
AFFERENT		
Medial Forebrain Bundle*	septal area reticular formation	lateral hypothalamus
Fornix	hippocampal formation	mammillary nucleus preoptic region
Stria Terminalis	amygdala	ventromedial region
Mammillotegmental Tract	midbrain	mammillary nuclei
Dorsal Longitudinal Fasciculus Central Tegmental Tract*	periaqueductal grey raphe nuclei	medial and posterior region
EFFERENT		
Medial Forebrain Bundle*	lateral hypothalamus	septal area reticular formation
Mammillothalamic Tract	mammillary nuclei	anterior n. thalamus
Mammillotegmental Tract	mammillary nuclei	reticular formation, midbrain and pons
Dorsal Longitudinal Fasciculus Central Tegmental Tract	medial and posterior region	reticular formation, entire brainstem
Neurohypophyseal Tract	tuberal region	posterior pituitary

*pathways with both afferent and efferent fibers

Review Exercises

15-1. Painful stimuli can produce brief bursts of adrenocorticotropic hormone (ACTH) from the anterior pituitary, even in a patient under general anesthesia. Considering that most general anesthetics block transmission from the thalamus to the cerebral cortex, suggest possible neural pathways and cellular regions which could be involved in this homeostatic response to pain.

15-2. Justify the observation that complete autonomic deafferentiation of the gut, while causing acute dysfunction, does not normally cause chronic dysfunction.

15-3. Refer to Patient #4 in the Appendix. When required to exercise, the patient shows an increase in heart rate of 5 to 10 bpm and either no change or a moderate decrease in systemic blood pressure (both systolic and diastolic). Explain these observations on the basis of the available and lacking autonomic connections between exercise response integration centers in the cortex, diencephalon and brainstem, and peripheral effectors such as the heart and peripheral vascular smooth muscle.

16

Homeostatic Regulation

The following classes of regulation with particular clinical relevance for the physical therapist will be considered:
1. Cardiovascular system regulation.
2. Regulation of the lung.
3. Temperature regulation.
4. Energy metabolism regulation.
5. Fluid balance regulation.
6. Diurnal cycling.

Cardiovascular System Regulation

Central neural components primarily involved in cardiovascular system regulation are located predominantly in the medulla (Fig. 16-1). The involved nuclei include the nucleus tractus solitarius (nTS) receiving relevant sensory information from baroreceptors (aortic by way of the vagus, carotid by way of the glossopharyngeal nerve) and atrial volume receptors (by way of the vagus). Additional cardiovascular sensory information is delivered to the adjacent reticular formation through spinoreticular fibers with sympathetic input. Interposed functionally between the cells of the nTS and the preganglionic motor control cells of the autonomic nervous system are several cell groups in the medullary reticular formation. These can be divided functionally into a dorsolateral pressor and a ventromedial depressor group. Evidence exists that integration of pressor and depressor signals occurs either in the preganglionic cells of the dorsal motor nucleus of the vagus or in the premotor interneurons in both the brainstem (parasympathetic) and spinal cord (sympathetic). A similar situation may exist for the sympathetic preganglionic neurons in the spinal cord. Sympathetic preganglionic cells innervating both the myocardium and vascular smooth muscle are innervated by way of descending reticulospinal fibers. The cyclic activity of the pressor and depressor cells is to a large extent self-generated, but it is definitely modulated both by incoming sensory information and by descending signals from higher levels in the neuraxis, particularly the cerebellum, the hypothalamus, and the cerebral cortex. The

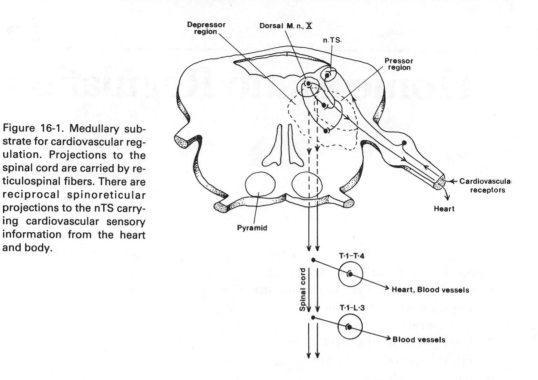

Figure 16-1. Medullary substrate for cardiovascular regulation. Projections to the spinal cord are carried by reticulospinal fibers. There are reciprocal spinoreticular projections to the nTS carrying cardiovascular sensory information from the heart and body.

sensory information is used to modulate the rate and amplitude of the basic control cycles.

At a lower level, cardiovascular reflex behavior can occur on the basis of spinal reflex pathways involving only the sympathetic system. Reflexes involving the heart are organized in the upper four thoracic segments; spinal reflex control of vascular smooth muscle can occur at all spinal levels containing sympathetic neurons. The importance of these spinal reflex circuits in the intact subject are not known. In the isolated spinal cord they sometimes appear to support positive rather than negative feedback behavior; however, in the intact person the characteristics of the spinal cardiovascular reflexes may be just the opposite. At both medullary and spinal levels, cardiovascular control is concerned primarily with the production of stereotyped reflex responses to sensory information concerning the state of the cardiovascular system. Integration between cardiovascular and respiratory behavior probably also occurs at the level of the medulla, indicating the very close reflex connections between these two systems.

Descending control from higher levels of the neuraxis appears necessary to provide integration of cardiovascular behavior with that of other homeostatic or somatomotor systems. Projections from the hypothalamus are essential for developing patterns of cardiovascular system activity supportive of various states, such as eating, exercising, or staying warm. More or less direct projections from the cerebral hemispheres probably are involved in making precise adjustments in these patterned or stereotyped behaviors.

The myocardium is innervated through parasympathetic preganglionic fibers carried in the vagus nerve to the cardiac plexus and sympathetic postganglionic fibers innervated from the first through the fourth thoracic spinal levels (Fig. 16-2).

Regulation of the Lung

In many ways, the substrate for regulation of breathing parallels that for the cardiovascular system, even to the extent of using the same nuclei and projection pathways. There is a definite possibility that at medullary and

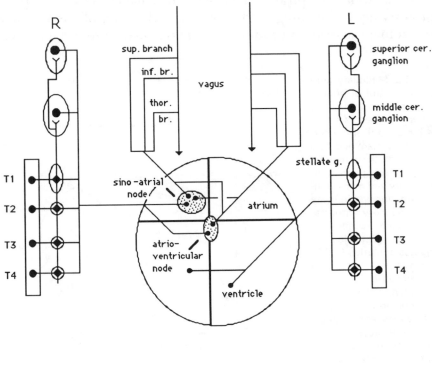

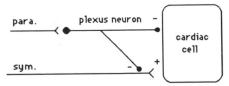

Figure 16-2. Sympathetic and parasympathetic innervation of the myocardium. Note the asymmetrical innervation: The right side of the sympathetic system innervates predominantly the pacemaker regions while the left side innervates predominantly the contractile muscle. Parasympathetic innervation is particularly important for the pacemaker regions and is essentially symmetrical. Within the cardiac plexus parasympathetic fibers can modify the behavior of the sympathetic system through presynaptic modification of synaptic activity. In this illustration the negative signs indicate synaptic activity which serves to inhibit either the cardiac cell or the sympathetic neuron.

higher levels some cells receive and integrate both cardiovascular and respiratory sensory information. Sensory information from chemoreceptors is delivered to the nTS over the vagus and glossopharyngeal nerves, with the addition of an intramedullary path from the ventral medullary chemoreceptors. Lung irritant and mechanoreceptor information is transmitted to the nTS by way of both the vagus and the ascending reticulospinal pathways (Fig. 16-3).

Control of lung function must act through both somatomotor and autonomic control systems. Neurons involved in somatomotor control are located within the medullary reticular formation. Inspiratory neurons are located dorsolaterally, and expiratory neurons located ventromedially. Additional reticular neurons located in the caudal pons have a predominantly inhibitory input to medullary inspiratory neurons. The balance between expiratory and inspiratory activity is integrated probably at the level of the motor neurons. The automatic activation produced by the reticular system can be over-ridden

Figure 16-3. Medullary substrate for control of breathing. The same areas of the brainstem are used as are involved in control of the cardiovascular system and, to a certain extent, there may be convergent projection of both sensory and motor control information within these regions. Sensory information from chemoreceptors is projected to the nucleus of the tractus solitarius *(n.TS.)* via the vagus (X) and from the chemosensory region in the ventral medulla. Sensory information from the chest wall (muscles and connective tissue) is projected over spinoreticular pathways *(sp.Ret. tr.).* Control signals are generated within the inspiratory and expiratory regions of the medullary reticular formation. Additional reticular formation control, inhibitory to breathing, is projected from the pontine reticular formation. Control of the muscles of breathing is projected over reticulospinal pathways to the diaphragm via the phrenic nerve and to the accessory muscles of breathing via their appropriate segmental nerves.

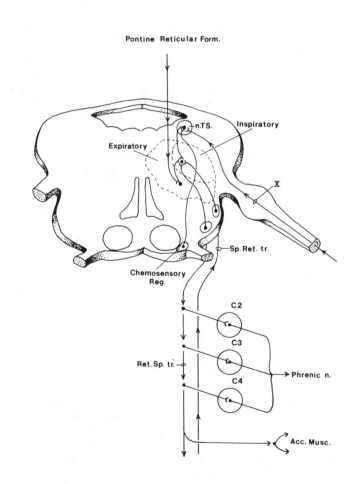

by voluntary control initiated in the cerebral cortex; the descending pathways for voluntary activation bypass the reticular system but send collaterals to it. The somatomotor outflow pathway consists primarily of the neurons of the phrenic nerve (C_2-C_4) to the diaphragm, plus motor neurons to other inspiratory and expiratory muscles (Fig. 16-3).

Control of activity of bronchial smooth muscle and the secretory epithelium of the larger airways also is integrated in the meduallary reticular formation. Parasympathetic preganglionic neurons are located in the dorsal motor nucleus of the vagus, and sympathetic preganglionic neurons are located in the upper thoracic intermediolateral horn (Fig. 16-3).

The cyclic behavior of both cardiovascular and breathing control neurons is strongly influenced by both incoming and descending information, but persists, although decreased, in the absence of such signals. This suggests that either individual cells or cell groups function as oscillators or pacemakers or complementary cell groups regulate each other through reciprocal inhibition, forming a basic oscillating circuit.

Temperature Regulation

Temperature regulation involves the coordinated control of the cardiovascular system, the respiratory system, the fluid balance system, the metabolism (both in general and in specific tissues), and the somatomotor system. Body core temperature is sensed by cells in the anterolateral region of the hypothalamus. This region, like a number of other regions of the CNS adjacent to the ventricular spaces, has a vascular supply with capillary walls permitting easy exchange of constituents between the blood and the extracellular fluid of the CNS. Thermoreceptive cells in the anterolateral region of the hypothalamus are apparently similar to peripheral thermoreceptors in having tuning curves for temperature. Some of these central cells thus are particularly sensitive to temperature lower than normal; while others are sensitive to increases in core temperature. Integration of temperature information for the purposes of producing temperature regulatory commands may occur in the thermoreceptors themselves or more likely, in additional cells in the anterior and posterior lateral regions of the hypothalamus. The integrator cells additionally receive information from peripheral thermoreceptors by way of ascending spinoreticular and spinothalamic pathways with direct or secondary projections to the hypothalamus. Other systems and receptors involved in homeostasis also project to temperature control regions of the hypothalamus. Temperature regulation thus can be coordinated with other other homeostatic needs of the body. The anterior lateral region of the hypothalamus may also be particularly susceptible to the presence of pyrogens in the blood. The sensitivity may be a result of the ease of exchange of materials in this region. It is unknown which cells pyrogens act on, whether they directly affect sensitivity of thermoreceptors or modify the activity of integrating cells.

Thermoregulatory control signals affecting the autonomic and somatomotor systems are transmitted through the medial forebrain bundle and possibly the dorsal longitudinal fasciculus to the reticular formation. Additional signals are transmitted to the tuberal region of the hypothalamus where they act on the cells involved in the production of thyrotropin releasing hormone (TRH). The effects of thermoregulation on various tissues are outlined in Table 16-1. Opposing sterotyped activation patterns exist for temperature deviation in either direction.

Energy Metabolism Regulation

Changes in energy metabolism are particularly important for thermoregulation, as indicated above, and for supporting tissue growth or repair.

TABLE 16-1. Thermoregulatory Responses of Tissues

Response	Tissue Involved	Control Pathways
DECREASED CORE TEMPERATURE		
Decreased blood flow to the skin	vascular smooth muscle	reticulospinal tract from medullary reticular formation to sympathetic preganglionic neurons
Piloerection	piloerector muscles	reticulospinal tract from medullary reticular formation to sympathetic preganglionic neurons
Increased excitability of skeletal muscle flexor motorneurons (posture adjusted and maintained to a greater degree in flexion)		reticulospinal tract from medullary reticular formation to flexor alpha and gamma motorneurons
Shivering (increased cocontraction of trunk, proximal limb muscles and jaw muscles accompanied by tremor-like activation)	skeletal muscle	?
Increased metabolic rate	skeletal muscle (shivering) adipose tissue (and other?)	? thyroid hormone
INCREASED CORE TEMPERATURE		
Increased blood flow to the skin	vascular smooth muscle	reticulospinal tract from medullary reticular formation to sympathetic preganglionic neurons
Increased respiratory rate	muscles of respiration	reticulospinal tract from medullary reticular formation to alpha and gamma motorneurons of muscles of respiration
Thermoregulatory sweating	thermoregulatory sweat glands	reticulospinal tract from medullary reticular formation to sympathetic preganglionic neurons
Decrease in alpha motor neuron excitability (postural adjustment and maintenance favoring extension at all joints)	skeletal muscle	reticulospinal tract from medullary reticular formation to alpha and gamma motorneurons

Changes in metabolism affect the use of energy metabolism substrate and in turn, are affected by the intake of substrate. A simple reflex loop for governing energy metabolism and substrate intake is illustrated in Figure 16-4. The general level of availability of energy substrate can be sensed by determining the blood glucose level. Cells in the ventromedial hypothalamus appear to have this sensing ability and function as "glucostats." Additionally, food intake is regulated by activity of other ventromedial cells that act to decrease appetite and lateral hypothalamic cells that act to increase appetite. The changes in feeding behavior brought about by these cells are related not only to energy metabolism substrate levels but also to the emotional state of the person. Emotional regulation of appetite and thus eating is a very complex and individualized process. Additional control of appetite appears to arise from activation of the somatomotor system, as occurs during exercise.

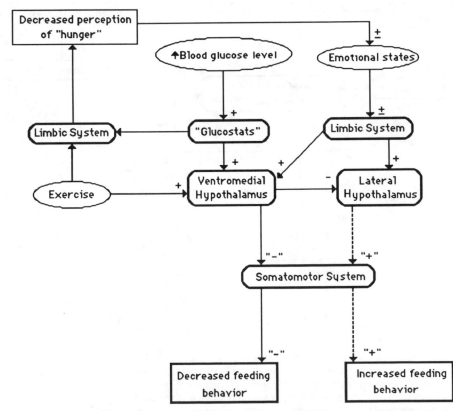

Figure 16-4. Negative feedback system governing energy metabolism and substrate intake. Both exercise and an increase in blood glucose level act on the control center in the ventromedial hypothalamus to produce a complex collection of commands resulting in decreased feeding behavior. Concurrently there is conscious perception of a decrease in hunger. This relatively simple system is complicated in unpredictable ways by the interaction between hunger and emotional states. The limbic system serves as the substrate to transmit emotion to the hypothalamus producing either an increase or a decrease in feeding behavior.

Fluid Balance Regulation

Sensory information that elicits changes in fluid balance regulation includes primarily the following (Fig. 16-5):

1. Central venous volume sensed by atrial and thoracic vein volume receptors.
2. Extracellular fluid osmolarity sensed by hypothalamic and renal osmoreceptors.

Additional regulatory information is derived from systemic and renal baroreceptors. The information from these receptors is integrated in or near the supraoptic nucleus of the hypothalamus. There are two separate response mechanisms to changes in extracellular fluid volume or osmolarity:

1. Altered renal function.
2. Altered drinking behavior.

Divergent projections from supraoptic and paraventricular cells releasing

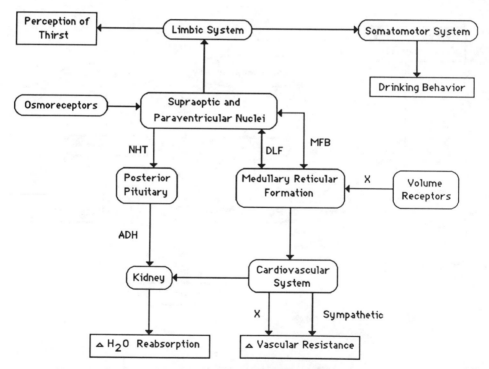

Figure 16-5. Negative feedback control system for fluid balance. Primary sensory input pathways involve osmoreceptors in the hypothalamus and volume receptors sending information to the medullary reticular formation. Integration of sensory information and generation of commands involves the supraoptic and paraventricular nuclei of the hypothalamus and the medullary reticular formation. Both neural and neurohormonal homeostatic control pathways are involved as well as somatomotor pathways. The resulting changes in behavior include the degree of water reabsorption by the kidneys, the extent of vascular resistance, and the presence of drinking behavior. The limbic system is the substrate involved in transmitting the sensory information to the level of conscious perception of thirst. *ADH,* antidiuretic hormone; *DLF,* dorsal longitudinal fasciculus; *MFB,* medial forebrain bundle; *NHT,* heurohypophyseal tract; *X,* vagus nerve.

antidiuretic hormone (ADH) may be responsible for both responses. One pathway from these nuclei projects to the posterior pituitary where ADH is released directly into the general circulatory system. Another pathway projects to the reticular formation by way of the medial forebrain bundle. Some fibers of this projection may continue into the spinal cord. The pituitary projections activate renal function adjustment. Brainstem and spinal projections may be responsible for supportive changes in cardiovascular system function through the autonomic nervous system. Hypothalamic projections to the limbic system are probably responsible for both the perception of thirst and the determination of the motor goal to seek something to drink.

A second aspect of fluid balance of considerable importance to the therapist is the storage and release of urine by the bladder. The bladder wall is composed of smooth muscle that receives both parasympathetic and sympathetic innervation (Fig. 16-6). Release of urine (micturition) is controlled also by contraction of the striated external sphincter and urogenital diaphragm muscles, which are innervated by somatomotor fibers in the pudic nerves. The micturition reflex is primarily a spinal reflex (Fig. 16-7). The lumbar sympathetic neurons provide excitatory input to the detrusor muscle; the sacral parasympathetic neurons excite the trigone and the internal sphincter of the bladder. Additionally, the parasympathetic neurons provide presynaptic inhibition to the sympathetic neurons. While the bladder is filling, the sympathetic system is inhibited and the parasympathetic facilitated. Thus the detrusor is relaxed and the trigone (that acts to assist the sphincter) and the internal sphincter are contracted. During micturition the situation is reversed. Under normal circumstances, this spinal reflex, like all others, is modified and con-

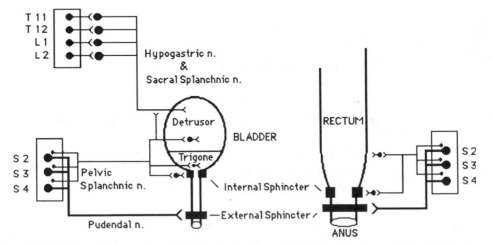

Figure 16-6. Pattern of innervation of the bladder and bowel. *Light lines,* autonomic innervation; *heavy lines,* somatomotor innervation. Parasympathetic innervation to the bladder from the sacral cord interacts with sympathetic innervation from the lumbar cord through both pre- and postsynaptic mechanisms within the bladder. There is no sympathetic innervation of the rectum and internal sphincter of the anus.

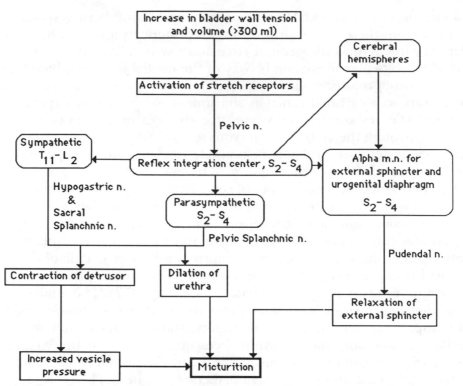

Figure 16-7. Flow diagram describing the micturition reflex. The primary system involves only the sacral integration center. The cerebral side loop permits voluntary override of the spinal reflex activity, as well as providing for coordinated activity in other voluntary muscles, such as those in the abdomen.

trolled by long loop projections to the cerebral hemispheres. The micturition reflex is a particularly good example of a close functional relationship between autonomic and somatomotor systems. A similar control system exists for the bowel.

This review of control of various homeostatic functions strongly suggests that there is divergent processing of commands enlisting the activity of many systems in each type of function. Possible substrate for this divergence includes primarily the extensive interconnections among hypothalamic nuclei and the brainstem reticular formation nuclei. Through these networks, sensory information specific to one function can be sent to a number of control centers, and patterned response behavior can be generated that interrelates the activity of most systems.

Diurnal Cycling

All of the homeostatic behaviors described, as well as most others, demonstrate cyclic peaks and valleys in activity level. For many homeostatic systems this cycling is diurnal or circadian, that is, it follows a twentyfour hour period. As is obvious, alterations in states of consciousness between sleep and waking also cycle with a twentyfour hour period. Determination of cause and effect relationships among behaviors demonstrating diurnal cycling is extremely difficult under normal circumstances. The identification of the behavior which is the pacemaker and those behaviors which are entrained by the pacemaker is not simple. Experiments have been conducted under circumstances where the subject is completely isolated from all external cyclic pacemakers such as natural light, social activity and clocks and calendars. Generally speaking the results indicate that 1) individuals have unique natural cycling periods and 2) distinct, non-circadian periods develop for various homeostatic behaviors in the absence of diurnally-varied stimuli.

The substrate involved in producing cyclic behavior clearly includes both the brainstem reticular formation and various hypothalamic nuclei. A pathway which has been suggested for bringing external diurnal stimuli into the hypothalamus and reticular formation involves optic nerve fiber projections to the suprachiasmatic nucleus of the hypothalamus (see Chapter 17). The importance of this pathway which transmits information on both light intensity and light quality is reflected in studies showing significant alterations in diurnal cycles in the absence or disruption of normal environmental light cycles.

Review Exercises

16-1.   Refer to Patient #2 in the Appendix. While the patient was in coma he required external intervention to control micturition (insertion of a catheter). He did not require a respirator to control breathing. Explain.

16-2.   Refer to Patient #4 in the Appendix. For one month following injury this patient demonstrated orthostatic hypotension (decrease in systemic blood pressure upon assuming the upright position). Explain. With gradual and consistent stimulation on a tilt table he was able to regain the ability to maintain a functional systemic blood pressure while upright. On the basis of what you know about central nervous system regeneration and about learning (synaptic plasticity) suggest some reasons for this return of normal reflex function.

16-3.   Refer to Patient #3 and Patient #4 in the Appendix. Both patients demonstrated persistent difficulty in regulating core body temperature during the rehabilitation phase of their treatment. Identify for each the most probable location of lesions affecting this aspect of homeostatic regulation, and the nuclei and/or tracts which are involved.

16-4.   Refer to Patient #4 in the Appendix. This patient eventually developed a hyperactive or spastic bladder with the inability to retain more than 100 cc of urine. Spinal cord injury patients with lesions in the lumbar region more typically develop hypotonic bladders. Discuss the reasons for these differing responses to spinal cord injury on the basis of your understanding of the relevant control pathways for micturition.

17

Vision and Visuomotor Behavior

Visual system function can be grouped into three main, interconnected categories:

1. Discriminatory use of visual sense information.
2. Non-discriminatory use of visual sense information.
3. Motor reflex use of visual sense information.

Discriminatory use of visual information includes all of those functions involved in conscious perception of vision such as color and form discrimination, spatial relationships among objects, and visual recognition of objects and patterns of movement. The substrate for these functions is predominantly cortical. Nondiscriminatory use of visual information involves adjustment of homeostatic functions in relation to the level of illumination, as for example in the generation of cyclic behavior entrained to a light-dark cycle. Substrate for these functions is predominantly subcortical, involving mainly the hypothalamus, the epithalamus, the autonomic nervous system, and the pituitary hormonal systems. Visuomotor reflexes involve adjusting the position of the head and eyes and the state of the various smooth muscles of the eyes to optimize reception of specifically attended visual stimuli. The anatomical components used in visuomotor reflexes of various types are extensive, involving both the cortex and the brainstem.

Anatomical Substrate Common to All Visual Functions

The eye and optic nerve are used to bring visual information to the point where it can be used for any general visual function (Fig. 17-1). The eye contains two functional components: 1) the retina with visual receptors and neurons with which they make connection and 2) the smooth and striated muscles used to adjust receptor function. The retina differs from other receptors, with the exception of olfactory cells, in being developmentally a part of the CNS (telencephalon). Retinal receptors are organized spatially in

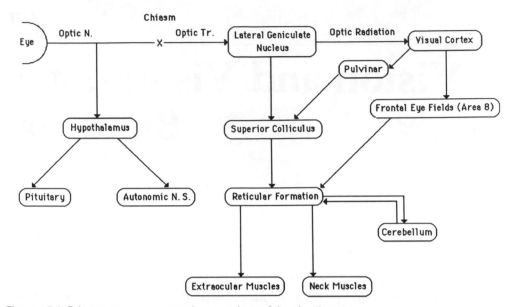

Figure 17-1. Primary components and connections of the visual system.

such a way that there is a gradation of function from the outer rim of the retina to the center (macula). The peripheral receptors (rods) are sensitive particularly to differences in light intensity and to movement of visual stimuli. They have relatively large receptive fields and are thus limited in their ability to discriminate stimulus boundaries precisely. Receptors in the macula (cones) are particularly sensitive to differences in light frequency or wavelength, and as a result of their small receptive fields, they are able to discriminate boundaries with great precision. The graded intermingling of rods and cones between the periphery and the macula, and the gradual shrinking of receptive fields of rods as they come closer to the macula, account for the smooth gradation in receptive capability of the retina.

Visual Fields

The space that can be seen by each retina is called the visual field, or the receptive field for the retina. As a result of the optics of the lens and cornea, objects in the visual field are projected on the retina in inverted fashion. The topographic mapping of the visual field on the retina is the basis for topographical projection of visual information for discriminatory purposes within the visual system. Topographic representation of visual space is maintained in all parts of the visuomotor system which use fine discrimination of object location (Fig. 17-2).

Components and Function of Discriminatory Vision

Discriminatory vision for the purposes of conscious identification and use of visual information involves processing of visual information within the occipital lobe (areas 17, 18, and 19) and projecting the processed information

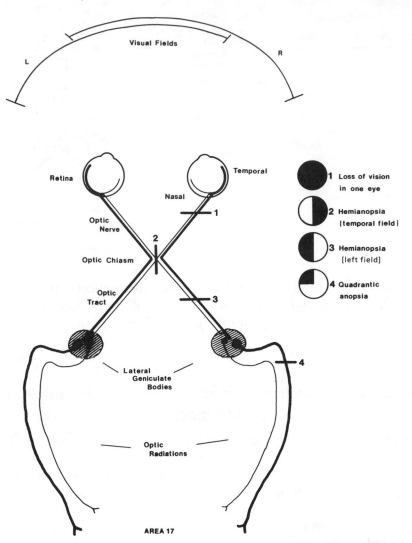

Figure 17-2. Projections of the visual fields within the visual system. The temporal portions of the retina of both eyes view overlapping central fields while the nasal retinas view separate lateral fields. Nasal retinal projections cross in the optic chiasm, permitting projection of an entire, contralateral visual field to each primary visual cortical hemisphere (area 17). Lesions of the visual projection system at the locations indicated will cause loss of projection of specific portions of the visual field as indicated in the circles on the right.

to specific regions of the temporal and parietal lobes (Fig.17-3). Processing of visual information within the temporal lobe appears to be related to attachment of meaning to visualized objects and involves convergent synaptic processing of information both from other sense systems and from the memory systems in the temporal lobe and hippocampus (part of the limbic system). Within the parietal lobe, visual information is processed in various ways, as directed by the needs of the person, to abstract specific types of information from the basic visual stimuli. The directing of these abstraction processes almost certainly involves projections to the parietal lobe from the frontal lobe

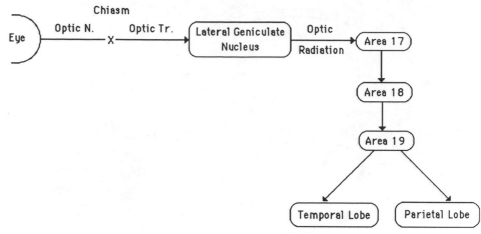

Figure 17-3. Substrate for discriminatory, perceptual use of visual information.

and the limbic system. The abstracted visual information can be used either for intellectual functions or for the direction of motor behavior related to vision. Commissural exchange of information from the primary visual cortex is essential for complete temporal and parietal lobe processing of the entire visual field.

Substrate and Function Related to Non-Discriminatory Visual Information

Some retinal neurons project directly (or possibly by collaterals) to the suprachiasmatic nucleus of the hypothalamus (Fig. 17-4). This nucleus is located immediately superior to the optic chiasm. Fibers projecting from this nucleus go to the habenular nucleus and probably the pineal body of the epithalamus. Both hypothalamic and epithalamic projections then go to the reticular formation of the brainstem and make diffuse connections with neurons involved in the development of cycles in homeostatic behavior. Shorter projections from the suprachiasmatic nucleus also terminate in other hypothalamic nuclei, influencing homeostatic behavior at this level of the neuraxis. Additional projections, not yet well defined, carry nondiscriminatory visual information to the limbic system where it can have an effect on the emotional state or mood of the individual. Within the nondiscriminatory visual system, the information provided concerns intensity and probably quality of the illumination. Topographic representation of the visual field is not maintained in this part of the visual system.

Visuomotor Substrate

There are three basic classes of visuomotor behavior, all of which function to optimize the projection of desired visual information on appropriate regions of the retina:

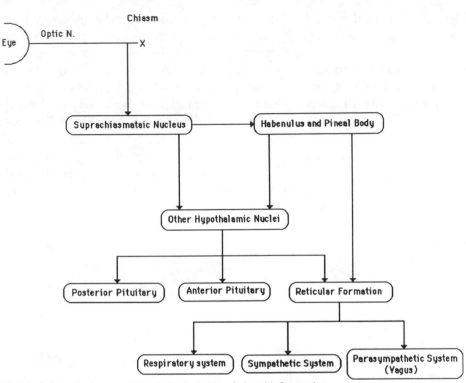

Figure 17-4. Substrate for non-discriminatory use of visual information.

1. Visual orienting, fixating, following, and exploratory movements of the eyes through the activation of the extraocular muscles.
2. Visual orienting, fixating, and following movements of the head through the activation of the neck muscles.
3. Adjustment of lens shape and pupillary diameter through the action of the ciliary muscle and pupillary sphincter.

Eye Movements

Activation of the extraocular muscles can accomplish the following adjustments of eye position:

1. Conjugate movement of both eyes, such that the visual image falls upon congruent portions of each retina.
2. Variable convergence of the eyes for flexible depth of focus.
3. Visual fixation on a stable object in the presence of head movement (optical righting of the eyes).
4. Visual tracking of an object moving across the visual field.
5. Saccades for the purpose of either visual exploration or rapid adjustment of the point of fixation for nonexploratory purposes (eg, reading).

The projection pathways supporting these extraocular muscle movements involve primarily the occipital lobe, the visual association regions in the parietal lobe, the frontal eye fields (area 8), the pulvinar (visual association nucleus in the thalamus), the superior colliculi and projections through the brainstem to the interstitial nucleus of Cajal adjacent to the oculomotor nucleus, the abducens nucleus, and the associated pontine reticular formation. From the interstitial nucleus of Cajal and the abducens nucleus, projections serving to coordinate activity in all the extraocular muscles are carried by the medial longitudinal fasciculus to cranial nerves III, IV and VI (Fig. 17-5). Elementary orienting eye movements can be generated by direct projections from the optic nerve or the lateral geniculate body, to the superior colliculus and the reticular formation (Fig. 17-6). In addition, the more complex movements requiring more decision making involve various regions of the cortex, depending on the exact type of movement required.

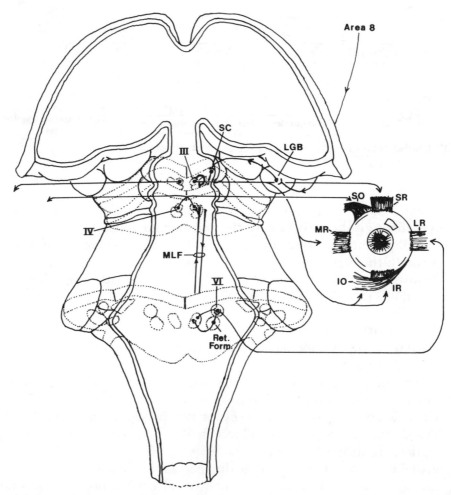

Figure 17-5. Basic visuomotor substrate. The pathways involved are very similar to those used for coordinating eye movement with vestibular sensory information. *IO,* internal oblique; *IR,* internal rectus; *LGB,* lateral geniculate body; *LR,* lateral rectus; *MLF,* medial longitudinal fasciculus; *MR,* medial rectus; *SC,* superior colliculus; *SO,* superior oblique; *SR,* superior rectus.

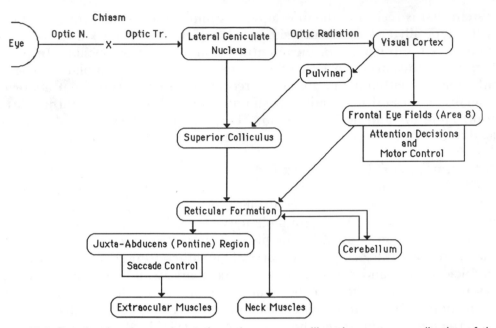

Figure 17-6. Functional pathways connecting substrate controlling visuomotor coordination of the extraocular and neck muscles. Note the two possible routes for transmission of visual information to the superior colliculus and reticular formation, and the involvement of the cerebellar side loop.

Neck movements that support visual orienting, tracking, and fixation involve essentially the same components as those for control of extraocular muscles, with the exception of control centers for saccadic type movements, which do not occur in neck muscles. Relevant visual information is projected to the superior colliculus either directly from the optic nerve or the lateral geniculate body or through more complex pathways involving the occipital and parietal lobes. Neck regions of areas 4 and 6 may be involved in the generation of visually-controlled neck movement, but area 8 is not involved (Fig. 17-6).

Movements of both the extraocular muscles and the neck in response to changing orientation of the visual field on the retina normally are congruent with the muscle activation that would be caused by vestibular stimulation occurring simultaneously. Thus, both optokinetic and vestibular nystagmus during rotation will move the eyes in the same direction. Visual righting reflexes, like vestibular righting reflexes, act on neck muscles in such a way as to return the head to an upright, eyes horizontal position. For this reason, the status of vestibular reflexes must always be evaluated with the eyes closed so that there will be no interaction available from the visual system. In situations where visual and vestibular information is not congruent (such as during the immediate postrotatory state or when on a ship or some types of amusement park rides),control of the extraocular and neck muscles comes under the dominance of the system to which the subject is directing attention or the system that is receiving the most intense stimulation. Normal congruent control is typically lacking in such situations, and functional neck and eye movements for the purposes of meaningful vision may not be possible. In pathological circumstances, a lack of congruence between vestibular and visual information, either from abnormal reception of stimuli or from abnormal interpretation and integration of stimuli, can lead to extreme difficulties in controlling eye and head orientation. This control problem can subsequently lead to difficulties in control of movement throughout the body.

Adjustments of the Lens and Pupil

The smooth muscles controlling lens shape and pupil diameter and the involuntary striated muscles controlling elevation of the upper eyelid are under the control of the autonomic nervous system (Fig. 17-7). Parasympathetic innervation is provided by fibers from the Edinger-Westphal nucleus that run with the oculomotor nerve. Sympathetic innervation arises from thoracic levels 1 and 2, with postganglionic fibers ascending from the cervical sympathetic ganglia to join the ophthalmic branch of the trigeminal nerve. Activation of these autonomic controls in response to visual stimuli can involve both the hypothalamus and the cerebral cortex (Fig. 17-8). Adjustment of lens

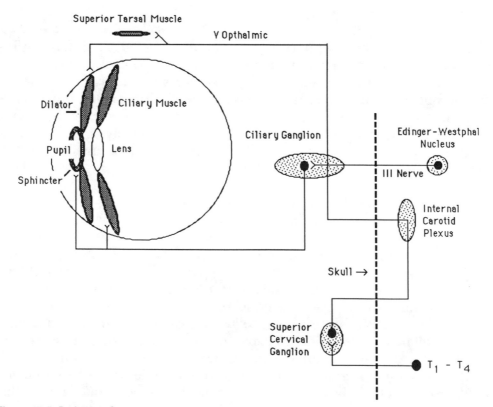

Figure 17-7. Pathways for autonomic innervation of intrinsic eye muscles.

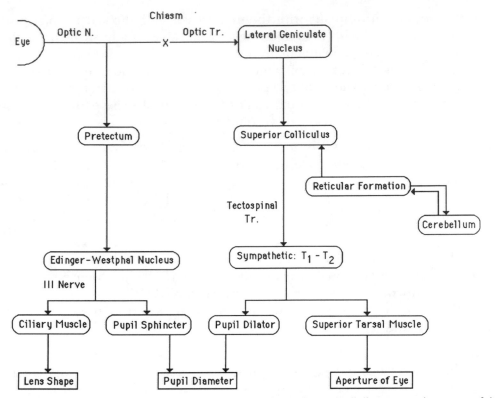

Figure 17-8. Substrate and connections for regulation of lens shape, pupil diameter and aperture of the eye.

shape is involved in focusing for near or distant objects in the visual field. Adjustment of pupillary diameter and upper eyelid position regulates the intensity of the illumination directed onto the retina. Adjustment of illumination intensity does not require discriminatory visual function and can operate without cortical input. Adjustment of focus requires cortical decision making. Both functions are organized in numerous small nuclei located in the pretectal region of the midbrain. Bilateral control of the lens and the pupil is enabled by exchange of information through the posterior commissure of the diencephalon. Due to the exclusive involvement of the midbrain in controlling the pupils, evaluation of pupil diameter and reflex adjustment is a useful tool in determining normalcy of midbrain structure and function.

Review Exercises

17-1. Refer to Patient #2 and Patient #3 in the Appendix. Both patients exhibited deficits in maintaining sitting balance. M.J. was completely lacking postural adjustment and posture maintenance responses in the left extremities and in the left axial muscles with or without visual input. She demonstrated normal post-rotatory nystagmus. E.G. demonstrated relatively normal postural adjustment movements with the eyes closed and showed normal post-rotatory nystagmus. With eyes open he was not able to adjust his body to a normal upright position or maintain it upright. On the basis of this information, and all other information you currently know about these patients, identify the most likely locations in either (or both) the visuomotor or vestibular motor response systems. Would you expect either of these patients to show any *perceptual* deficits for visual or vestibular information?

17-2.   Refer to Patient #3 in the Appendix. Upon admission following the initial trauma E.G. demonstrated an ipsilateral pupillary light reflex (constriction) to light shone in the right eye. There was no consensual response in the left eye. There was no response in either eye to light shone in the left eye. What is the most likely *single* location of a lesion causing this particular pattern of response?

17-3.   In some individuals, winter is a time during which they experience clinical depression (seasonal affective disorder, SAD). The absence or limitation of what normal sensory stimulus may be involved? What pathways exist to bring this stimulus into the central nervous system and to project it to the limbic system and frontal association cortex?

17-4.   Generate a flow diagram, with the correct anatomical substrate identified, which describes the process by which increased muscle activity such as occurs during exercise elicits an increase in rate and depth of breathing.

17-5.   Physicians have been aware for some time of the importance of timing drug administration with regard to diurnal cycles. Identify some physical therapeutic interventions which typically have an impact on homeostatic functions such as thermoregulation, blood flow distribution, breathing patterns and fluid balance. What information concerning diurnal cycling of these behaviors could you use to maximize the beneficial effects of therapeutic intervention?

17-6.   Refer to Patient #2 in the Appendix. This patient demonstrates left hemianopsia. (Hemianopsia is a loss of half of the total visual field.) What is the most likely *single* location of a lesion causing this problem?

18

Limbic System

Anatomically, the limbic system comprises the oldest part of the cerebral hemispheres and associated structures in the diencephalon and midbrain. Generally speaking, the cortical structures associated with the limbic system have developed from parts of the rhinencephalon, the part of the brain originally related to olfactory function (Fig. 18-1). Humans use the sense of smell relatively little, and most of the rhinencephalon has developed the ability to process information from all senses. The two principal archicortical limbic structures, which are the cingulate gyrus and the hippocampal formation, form a nearly complete circle deep in the cerebral hemispheres in close association with the lateral ventricles. They are joined by axons projecting from the cingulate gyrus to the hippocampal formation in the induseum griseum (longitudinal striae) just external to the corpus callosum. The remaining cortical components of the limbic system are located in the ventral portion of the frontal lobe (orbital gyri, subcallosal area, paraterminal gyrus) and the temporal lobe (parahippocampal gyrus containing the entorhinal cortex). The hooked tip of the temporal lobe, or uncus, contains a subcortical or deep nuclear component of the limbic system: the amygdala. The septal nuclei of the septum pellucidum may also be considered part of the limbic system, although they are sometimes included with the hypothalamus. The limbic cortex communicates with a number of hypothalamic nuclei but most directly with the mammillary bodies. The thalamic nuclei acting as specific relay nuclei for the limbic system are the anterior and dorsomedial nuclei. Additional cellular structures related to the limbic system include the habenulus in the epithalamus and the interpeduncular nuclei of the midbrain that are associated with the reticular formation. The cellular structures of the limbic system are summarized in Table 18-1.

The major fiber pathways of the limbic system can be grouped into four categories: curved pathways that are to a certain extent functionally bidirectional, ventral pathways, pathways through the thalamus, and limbic system commissures. The curved pathways more of less closely follow the anterior to posterior curve of the lateral ventricle. Ventral pathways primarily provide

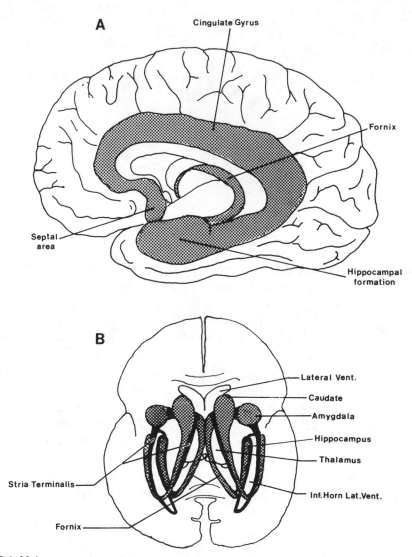

Figure 18-1. Main components of the limbic system. A. Midsaggital view showing the cingulate gyrus in the frontal and parietal lobes, the septal region in the frontal lobe, the hippocampal formation in the temporal lobe, and the fornix. B. Dorsal view showing the relationships of C-curved structures related to the lateral ventricles.

connections between temporal lobe components of the limbic system and hypothalamic or frontal lobe components. There are several commissures involving the limbic system, primarily the anterior commissure connecting temporal lobes and passing through the septal region, the commissural fibers of the fornix (a major curved pathway), and the habenular commissure connecting the two habenular nuclei of the epithalamus. The major pathways used by the limbic system and their connections are summarized in Table 18-2.

The primary function of the limbic system appears to be collecting and

TABLE 18-1. Cellular Components of the Limbic System

Component	Location
Hemispheric Structures	
Subcallosal and Paraterminal Gyri	frontal lobe, ventral to genu of corpus callosum
Orbital Gyri	frontal lobe, ventral surface (dorsal to orbits)
Septal Nuclei	septum pellucidum
Cingulate Gyrus	frontal and parietal lobes adjacent to corpus callosum
Hippocampal Formation · hippocampus · parahippocampal gyrus · dentate gyrus	temporal lobe medial to inferior horn of the lateral ventricle
Amygdala	uncus of temporal lobe, anterior to tip of the inferior horn of the lateral ventricle
Diencephalic and Mesencephalic Structures	
Mammillary Bodies	posterior ventral hypothalamus
Anterior Nuclear Group of Thalamus	anterior thalamus
Dorsomedial Nucleus of Thalamus	dorsal thalamus
Habenular Nucleus	epithalamus
Interpeduncular Nucleus	midbrain tegmentum, dorsomedial to cerebral peduncles

TABLE 18-2. Primary Limbic Fiber Pathways

Tract	Connections	
Curved Pathways		
Induseum Griseum (longitudinal striae)	cingulate gyrus	parahippocampal gyrus (entorhinal cortex)
Fornix	hippocampus	· septal region · hypothalamus (general) · mammillary bodies
Stria Terminalis	amygdala	· septal region · hypothalamus (general)
Stria Medullaris	septal region	habenular nucleus
Ventral Pathways		
Ventral Amygdalofugal Pathway	amygdala	hypothalamus (general)
Medial Forebrain Bundle	olfactory tubercle	septal region
Habenulopeduncular Tract	habenulus	interpeduncular nuclei
Thalamic Pathways		
Mammillothalamic Tract	mammillary bodies	anterior nucleus of thalamus
Internal Capsule (anterior limb and genu)	· anterior nucleus of thalamus	cingulate gyrus
	· dorsomedial nucleus of thalamus	frontal association cortex
Limbic Commissures		
Anterior Commissure	anterior temporal lobe	anterior temporal lobe
Fornix	hippocampus	hippocampus
Habenular Commissure	habenular nucleus	habenular nucleus

processing sensory and association cortical information and returning it to the association cortex by way of the hypothalamus. There are two main processing loops, one involving the cingulate gyrus and hippocampal formation and the other involving the amygdala (Fig. 18-2). Information enters the limbic system through one of three entry regions: the cingulate gyrus, the parahippocampal gyrus, or the amygdala. The cingulate gyrus collects information from the entire frontal and parietal lobes and in turn projects either to the parahippocampal gyrus over the induseum griseum (longitudinal stria) or to the amygdala over ventral pathways in the frontal lobe. Information from the occipital lobe either may enter the cingulate gyrus after being processed in the parietal lobe or may enter the parahippocampal gyrus after processing in the temporal lobe. Most of the association cortex of the temporal lobe projects to the parahippocampal gyrus. Olfactory information in the anterior portion of the temporal lobe and the orbital region of the frontal lobe may project into either the amygdala or the parahippocampal gyrus.

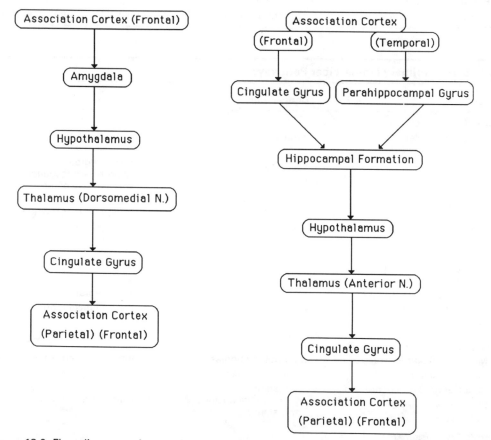

Figure 18-2. Flow diagrams of transmission of information in the two main limbic processing loops. *Left,* the loop through the amygdala. *Right,* the loop through the hippocampal formation. Although both loops both begin and end in association cortex, different regions of the association cortex are involved.

The hippocampal formation is located in the ventromedial portion of the temporal lobe immediately medial to the inferior horn of the lateral ventricle. It contains the dentate gyrus and its surrounding hippocampus (Fig. 18-3). Hippocampal afferent fibers reach the dentate gyrus from the entorhinal cortex of the adjacent, more medially placed parahippocampal gyrus. Afferent projections to the entorhinal cortex arise from both the cingulate gyrus and the olfactory regions of the temporal lobe. Efferent hippocampal projections arise from pyramidal cells in the three-layered hippocampal cortex and are collected into two fiber bundles: the lateral alveus and medial fimbria of the hippocampus. These fiber bundles combine to form the fornix. The fornix transmits hippocampal output information to various areas of the hypothalamus, including the mammillary bodies. Some fornix fibers are also commissural, providing a link between the hippocampal formation in both hemispheres. The fornix is also capable of carrying information from the hypothalamus back to the hippocampal formation. The limbic circuit involving the hippocampus is completed through mammillary projections to the

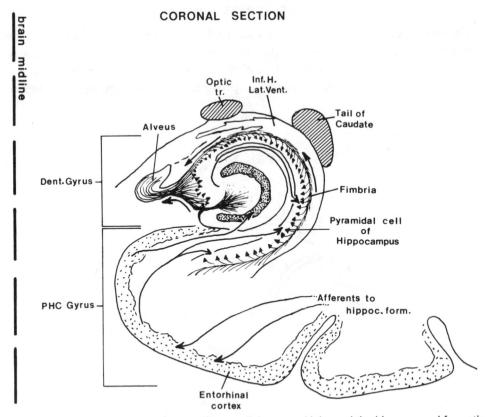

Figure 18-3. Coronal section through the ventromedial temporal lobe and the hippocampal formation. The primary pathway through the hippocampus involves afferent fibers to the entorhinal cortex of the parahippocampal gyrus *(PHC Gyrus).* Fibers from this region project to the dentate gyrus within the hippocampus. The efferent cells of the hippocampus are the pyramidal cells which project their fibers into the fimbria and the alveus which together form the fornix.

anterior nucleus of the thalamus that in turn projects through the internal capsule to the cingulate gyrus. The principal circuit through the cingulate gyrus, hippocampus, and anterior nucleus of the thalamus is shown schematically in Figure 18-4.

Unlike the hippocampal formation that collects most of its cortical information from the cingulate gyrus, the amygdala collects cortical input directly from the orbital cortex of the frontal lobe and from the association cortex in the temporal lobe. Like the hippocampal formation, it also derives afferents from the septal region and the hypothalamus, but by way of the stria terminalis rather than the fornix. The efferent projections from the amygdala basically reciprocate the afferent input (Fig. 18-5). The predominant efferent connection is to the hypothalamus by way of the stria terminalis. Additional hypothalamic projections are carried by the ventral amygdalofugal pathway. The dorsomedial nucleus of the thalamus serves as the specific relay nucleus for the amygdala, transmitting information received from various hypothalamic nuclei to the frontal association cortex.

Limbic System Function

The limbic system appears to be essential for two related and more or less conscious processes: 1) establishing emotional states or mood on the basis of current or recalled information and 2) attaching meaning or value to sensory information. It may also be of major importance in establishing a link between

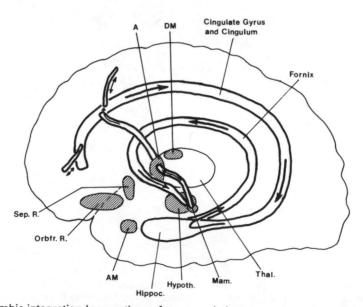

Figure 18-4. Limbic integration loop pathway from association cortex through the cingulate gyrus, to the hippocampal formation via the cingulum, to the hypothalamus via the fornix, to the anterior nucleus of the thalamus via the mammillothalamic tract, and returning to the association cortex via the anterior limb of the internal capsule and cingulate-cortical projections.

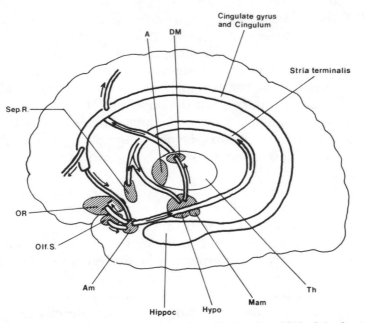

Figure 18-5. Limbic integration loop pathway from the orbital regions *(OR)* of the frontal lobe to the amygdala and from here to the hypothalamus and septal regions via the stria terminalis. The ventral amygdalofugal pathway to the hypothalamus is not shown. The return pathway to the cortex involves hypothalamic projections to the dorsomedial nucleus *(DM)* of the thalamus *(Th)* and internal capsule projections to the cingulate gyrus which then projects to the association cortex.

homeostatic needs and conscious behavior. These processes involve what is termed "meaning" memory, thus the limbic system is also one part of the CNS in which memory occurs.

The processing loop involving the cingulate gyrus and hippocampal formation was suggested by James Papez (1937) as a main pathway for the development of emotional states. Activity in this circuit is important for developing the motivation to do any particular act.

Evidence is growing that some affective psychological disorders may involve disruption of adrenergic and serotonergic transmission through the ventral limbic pathways, primarily the medial forebrain bundle. Schizophrenia, a thought disorder, may be caused in part by altered dopaminergic transmission from the midbrain to the orbital gyri.

Memory

Four basic types of memory have been described:
1. Identification memory: recall of the identification of specific sensory information.
2. Meaning memory: recall of the value or meaning of a bit of information.
3. Process memory: recall of the steps or procedure for sequencing a mental or motor activity.
4. Storytelling memory: ability to organize past events into a logical whole.

These different types of memory involve the use of different substrates within the CNS. Identification memory uses substrates within the temporal and parietal association cortex. Meaning memory involves the limbic system. Process memory can involve many wide-spread portions of the CNS. This type of memory for motor acts, for example, involves both the frontal association cortex and all of the components of the middle level of the motor hierarchy: motor cortex, basal ganglia, and cerebellum. Process memory for mental activity appears to involve various regions of the parietal and frontal association cortex. Storytelling memory also involves association cortex, primarily in the frontal and parietal lobes.

As a result of the dispersion of various types of memory to different cortical regions, isolated memory deficiencies can occur. When meaning memory is lost, a person may be able to identify an object but not use it appropriately. Loss of identification memory leads to inability to name or recognize objects. Its reliance on specific sensory input can be demonstrated in cases where a person may be able to recognize an object using one sensory modality but not another. Loss of process memory in relationship to motor activity leads to the problem of dyspraxia in which a person can clearly identify movement goals but cannot logically sequence motor behavior to reach the goal. With loss of storytelling memory, the person appears confused about the sequence or existence of past events.

The mechanisms through which memory develops are not specifically known. Memory pathways are almost certainly highly convergent, permitting an orderly association of one bit of information with others. On a time basis, all categories of memory can be divided into short-term and long-term memory. Short-term memory probably involves relatively transient changes in synaptic behavior such as posttetanic facilitation. Long-term memory probably requires additional structural changes in synapses that act to increase the security of specific convergent pathways. The dependence of memory on either repetition or intensity of information suggests that the synaptic changes are the result of trophic influences arising from the use of specific synapses.

The generation of emotional states and the use of memory are certainly functions that would be attributed to "mind." Even though definite progress has been made in identifying the anatomical substrate required for these functions and some of the synaptic behaviors that appear to be involved in producing them, there still is no clear determination of the constellation of neural substrates and functions through which a mechanistic but complex brain gives rise to a mind.

Olfactory System

The olfactory system is closely associated structurally, developmentally, and possibly functionally, with the limbic system. The main components of the olfactory system lie adjacent to the orbital gyri; their projections enter the septal region, orbital cortex, and entorhinal cortex (Fig. 18-6). Perhaps because of this anatomically direct relationship with the limbic system, olfaction is not only one of the least localized sensations but also one of the best at evoking complex memories.

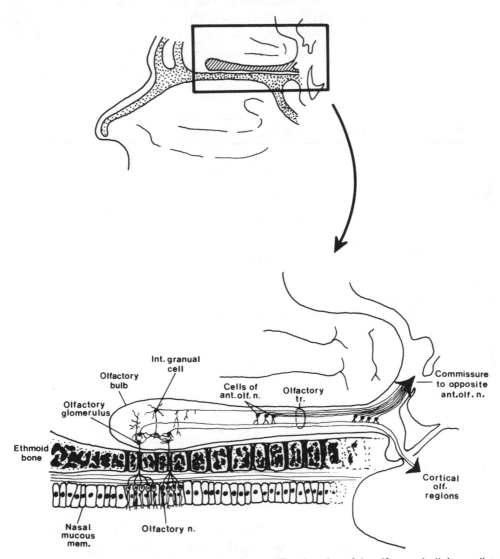

Figure 18-6. Major components of the olfactory system. *Top,* location of the olfactory bulb immediately dorsal to the cribiform plate of the ethmoid bone. *Bottom,* primary (olfactory neuron), secondary (internal granual cell) and tertiary (anterior olfactory nucleus) cells of the olfactory system. Interneurons within the olfactory bulb have the distinction of having no identified axons; they interact solely through dendritic and somatic synapses.

The primary afferents of the olfactory system have their cell bodies within the CNS, in the paired olfactory bulbs immediately superior to the cribiform plate of each nostril. Within the olfactory bulb there is synaptic provision for a large amount of information processing, including efferent control of synaptic activity. Second order olfactory neurons in the olfactory tract send projections to the anterior olfactory nucleus at the base of the tract. Third order projections carry olfactory information to the parahippocampal gyrus, the amygdala, and the orbitofrontal cortex on the side of entry, and to the olfactory bulb, on the opposite side, by way of the anterior commissure. Additional projections of olfactory information reach the hypothalamus and additional regions of the temporal lobe. Table 18-3 summarizes the components of the olfactory system.

Table 18-3. Cellular Components of the Olfactory System

Component	Location
Olfactory Neurons	
Primary	nasal mucosa
Secondary	olfactory bulb
Tertiary	anterior olfactory nucleus
Olfactory Integration Neurons	pyriform region of temporal lobe adjacent to hippocampal formation
Cortical Receptor Regions	
Parahippocampal Gyrus	temporal lobe
Orbitofrontal Cortex	frontal lobe
Subcortical Receptor Regions	
Amygdala	uncus of temporal lobe
Septal Region	hypothalamus

Review Exercises

18-1.   The mammillary bodies appear to have a major integration and relay function related to homeostasis. Describe possible pathways through the mammillary bodies which could translate the emotion of anxiety into an increase in heart rate and palmar sweating.

18-2.   Identify those parts of the central nervous system which are most likely to undergo synaptic modification during the process of learning and remembering the motor behavior of catching a ball.

18-3.   If you inserted a pin into the temporal lobe from the lateral side, in what order would you pass through the following structures:
- inferior horn of the lateral ventricle
- hippocampus
- superior temporal gyrus

- parahippocampal gyrus
- hypothalamus
- third ventricle

18-4. Structural Models: Due to the anatomical dispersion of the components of the limbic system in three planes it is difficult to generate a concept of their spatial relationships. Models can be made of:

a. any of the "C"-curved limbic pathways in relationship to the thalamus and the lateral ventricle
b. the ventral longitudinal diencephalic pathways
c. the limbic commissures and intra-hemispheric pathways lying in or near the horizontal plane.

19

Higher Cortical Functions

The primary sensorimotor regions of the cerebral hemispheres and the limbic cortex have already been identified and had their functions described. The association cortex, located in frontal, parietal, and temporal lobes, has four identified functions:

1. Abstraction and recombination of elements of primary sensory information from adjacent sensory regions, specifically:
   · parietal: visual, somatosensory, and auditory information, possibly including taste;
   · temporal: auditory and olfactory information; and
   · frontal: olfactory information.
2. Directed and flexible combination and interpretation of two or more major types of sensory information.
3. Generation of behavior patterns.
4. Generation of consciousness.

The substrate for the first two functions is becoming increasingly well defined, as are the synaptic behaviors bringing about these functions. Substrate and processes involved in the generation of behaviors also are becoming defined. The substrate and particularly the processes involved in the generation of conscious thought, or "mind," still is almost completely a matter of speculation, although many components of conscious functions have been localized to specific lobes.

The association region of the frontal lobe, also termed the prefrontal cortex, is involved in a number of conscious behaviors that appear to rely strongly on interaction with various portions of the limbic system. Behaviors depending on an intact prefrontal cortex (or its afferent and efferent connections) include the following:

1. Affective behavior: *expression* of emotions.
2. Adjustment of behavior to the social environment.

3. Imagination: abstraction and novel recombination of available information. May involve or be a location for storytelling memory.
4. Production of communication.

The temporal association cortex also relies extensively on connections with the limbic system for its functions. It is involved in the following:

1. Development of emotional states or mood (as distinct from expression of emotion).
2. Generation of a sense of humor.
3. Expression of sexual behavior.
4. Development of memory of various kinds, particularly identification and meaning memory.

The temporal association cortex functions in close association with the parietal association cortex in the process of understanding communication.

The parietal association cortex has major involvement in functions requiring integration of visual, auditory and somatosensory information. Primary functions include the following:

1. Various aspects of spatial organization of sensory information leading to the development of spatial orientation and the generation of a body image.
2. Logical ordering of sensory information including temporal sequencing.
3. Development of abstract and symbolic logic such as mathematical calculation and language.

Most of the functions described for association cortex do not require paired mirror-image lateralization of information such as is seen in the primary reception of sensory information or the immediate production of motor behavior. Indeed, most association cortex functions require either bilateral distribution of information or direction of information related to both sides of the body to only one hemisphere. A major function of the hemispheric commissures (corpus callosum and anterior commissure) thus is to provide a route for 1) exchange of sensory information among hemispheres to permit asymmetrical parallel processing of that information and 2) for exchange of the results of association cortex processing to permit production of coordinated motion bilaterally. Many association cortex functions thus can be localized in one hemisphere or the other and need not occur in both hemispheres. This has given rise to functional asymmetries in association cortex, which in some cases are clearly related also to structural asymmetries (Fig. 19-1). In most people the functions indicated are localized in a hemisphere dominant for that function; in some cases dominance is shared between the two hemispheres (eg, ambidextrousness). Major asymmetrically lateralized function include the following:

1. Motor behavior.
2. Communication.
3. Auditory perception.
4. Spatial perception.
5. Logical ordering of information.
6. Generation of emotional states.

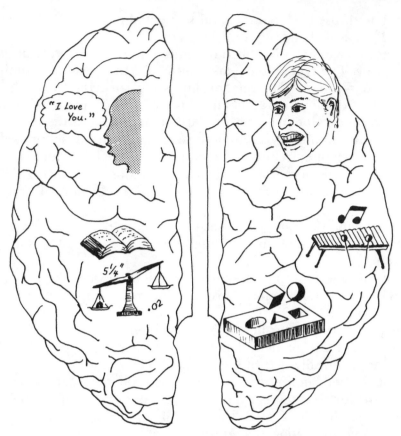

Figure 19-1. Typical asymmetrical localization of higher cortical functions.

Very generally speaking, the logic produced in processing of sensory information in the association cortex of the parietal and temporal lobes differs between the right and left hemispheres. The right hemisphere appears to produce parallel or holistic logic when processing information, whereas the left hemisphere appears to generate sequential logic. The sequential logic used by the left hemisphere gives rise to the ability to use syntactic rules for communication, to develop mathematical calculations, and to organize events in a temporal sequence. The parallel logic used in the right hemisphere permits spatial organization of sensory information and the development of symbolic and tonal communication. Differences in the ability to perceive auditory information support these deferences in logic. The left temporal lobe is important for perception of the sequence of auditory sensation, which is used as a basis for developing syntactic communication or language. The right temporal lobe is more capable of perceiving the tonal qualities of auditory sensation. The right parietal lobe has more facility than the left in processing visual or tactile information to produce recognition of objects based on their spatial organization or overall visual pattern. Although the two hemispheres produce different styles of logical organization of things and events, they both use both parallel and sequential processing of information (as opposed to parallel and sequential logic).

Hemispheric asymmetry has been recognized most clearly in relationship to motor behavior. The type of movement most affected by motor dominance is fractionated movement. This relationship is not surprising considering the complete lack of organizing centers for this type of movement below the level of the cortex. Motor dominance is predicated on the use of the extremities in coordinated, predominantly asymmetrical, patterns for fractionated movement. This pattern of extremity use requires all of the following:

1. An embryologic organization of anatomical substrate which gives preference to one hemisphere or the other for production of fractionated movement.
2. Development of learned or secure synaptic pathways for skilled or highly automatic movements, based on the presence of this anatomical asymmetry.
3. Communication through the corpus callosum between the frontal association cortex of both hemispheres leading to coordination of movement in opposite extremities.

The dominant motor hemisphere is determined initially by genetic programming. Subsequent use of neural pathways during development can either reinforce the genetically determined structural asymmetry or negate it to a large extent. Either hemisphere may be genetically designated as dominant for motor function, but there is a definite preponderance of left hemisphere dominance (right-handedness) in the general population.

There is some indication that development of emotional states also is a lateralized function. The left temporal association cortex appears essential for elevating mood; the right side is involved in depressing mood.

A certain level of correlation has been demonstrated between dominant hemispheres for motor behavior and sequential logic. This has been examined most precisely for syntactic language function and hand dominance. The correlation is not exact, which suggests either that genetic determination of dominance is separate for different association functions or that subsequent development can interact in unique ways with each cortical region.

Disturbances of cortical association function can be classed generally as involving sensory perception (agnosias), motor planning (dyspraxias or apraxias), or communication skills (dysphasias or aphasias). Agnosias are usually modality-specific. There is a loss of ability to recognize objects when they are presented to the involved sensory system, even when the ability to describe the sensory information is retained. A person with a pure visual agnosia, for example, might be able to describe what a spoon looked like but could not identify it as a spoon when seeing it. Upon handling the spoon, the person would be able to identify it. Agnosias typically are due to parietal or temporal lobe damage.

Apraxias are disturbances of motor planning, which may affect various aspects of motor planning and more or less limited sets of muscles. Examples of apraxias would include the following:

1. Correct recognition of an object but inability to use it appropriately.
2. Inability to sequence available movements into a normal pattern.
3. Inability to mimic movements.
4. Inability to produce movements on command.

Some types of apraxia may produce clumsy movements, but paresis or paralysis of movement is not involved. The association cortex in the parietal and upper temporal regions and in the frontal lobe have been implicated as sites for motor planning that can be disrupted in apraxia.

Communication

Disturbances of language or communication function are classed as aphasias. These disorders may involve either the reception or the production of communications. Communication involves three basic components:

1. Symbolic visuomotor or tactile-motor behavior.
2. Symbolic tone and rhythm.
3. Language.

All three of these components are used usually with complete congruence in any given communication. Communications become confused when there is a loss of congruence.

Visuomotor or tactile-motor communication is the production, reception, and interpretation of symbolic motor behavior. It involves mimetic use of facial muscles; gestures of the upper or lower extremities; and posture of the head, trunk, and extremities. Communication of this type most typically is received visually, but may also be received tactually when gestures involve touching. This type of communication has been formalized as dance and pantomime.

Tone and rhythm are involved in communication through attachment of symbolic meaning to specific tones or rhythms. Typically ,this aspect of communication is received through auditory sensation, although rhythm may be received tactually through mechanoreceptors. Although tone and rhythm are components of any language, they have varying degrees of importance in different languages. For example, the word "tree" in English means a relatively large plant with branches and leaves, no matter how you say it. A word with the same sound in Chinese might mean a number of very different things, depending on the tonal quality used in saying it.

Language is the production, reception, and interpretation of ordered symbolic vocalization (spoken language) that can be given specific visual (or tactile) form (written language). Language differs from the other components of communication by requiring sequential logic for its development and use. Language may be received equally well using visual, auditory, or tactile modalities.

The symbolic motor behavior and tonal components of communication appear to be lateralized to the right hemisphere. Language is associated typically with the left hemisphere; however, language dominance may occur in the right hemisphere. Language dominance frequently, but not always, is associated with motor dominance. As with motor dominance, in some cases language function is present bilaterally. The anatomical substrate for communication is essentially the same in both hemispheres, but portions of it are considerably enlarged in the language-dominant hemisphere.

Communication function is localized to specific regions of the association cortex in the temporal, parietal, and frontal lobes (Fig. 19-2). These cortical regions are connected by the arcuate fasciculus. The necessity for both specific sets of cells and the connections among them for complete normal language function was one of the major experimental proofs of the cellular connection theory of cortical function.

Wernicke's area in the temporal lobe is essential for the perception of communication received by the auditory system. Dejerine's area (angular gyrus) is involved in the perception of communication received over visual or tactile routes. Both Wernicke's and Dejerine's areas appear to be involved in the development of sequential logic necessary for the understanding and generation of language. Broca's area in the frontal lobe is used in the production of motor behavior involved in communication, whether it be gesture, vocalization, or writing. Commissural connections are necessary for transfer of either sensory information or motor plans to the appropriate hemisphere (Fig. 19-3).

To produce spoken language, there must be coordination among the movements of the jaw, tongue, lips, pharynx, and vocal cords and the activation of

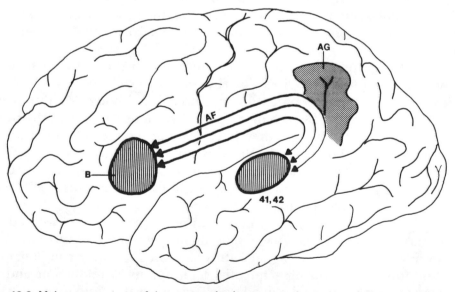

Figure 19-2. Major components of the communication system. Areas 41 and 42 are primary auditory receptor areas. The angular gyrus (AG) receives visual communication information and provides integration of visual and auditory information. The arcuate fasciculus (AF) connects these two areas with Broca's region (B) in the frontal lobe. Broca's region provides motor control for expressing communication. Transmission of information in the angular gyrus can be bidirectional, with the primary functional movement being that from the sensory areas toward the motor control area.

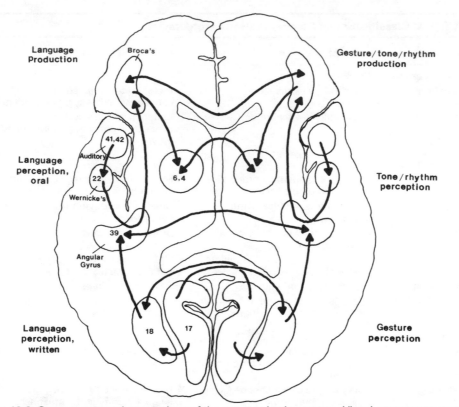

Figure 19-3. Components and connections of the communication system. Visual sensory communication is received in area 17 and further processed in area 18. Auditory sensory information is received in areas 41 and 42 and further processed in area 22 (Wernicke's region). The angular gyrus (area 39) receives processed visual and auditory communication information (and possibly tactile communication information as well). The arcuate fasciculus projects to Broca's area in the frontal lobe which controls production of communication, whether that be verbal or non-verbal. Projections from Broca's area to the premotor (6) and motor (4) areas provide commands for appropriate muscle activation. There is extensive commissural transmission of communication information through the corpus collosum at all points in this system.

the muscles of respiration. Broca's area thus must send projections to the portions of areas 6 and 4 involved in control of these sets of muscles. The necessary coordinating commands are carried from the motor cortex cortico-bulbar projections to the cranial nerves innervating the muscles of the mouth and to the medullary respiratory center and by corticospinal projections to respiratory motor neurons.

Clearly, many opportunities exist for disturbances of communication. These can be classified generally as "peripheral" language and "cortical" communication disorders or aphasias (Tab. 19-1). The peripheral disorders involve the sensorimotor coordination necessary to produce spoken language. *Dysarthria* is faulty articulation of words resulting from inadequate control of mouth muscles at some level. Orofacial dyspraxia may produce a type of dysarthria. *Dysphonia* is faulty vocalization or production of sound resulting

TABLE 19-1. Classification of Communication Disorders

Type	Symptoms	Location of Lesion
Peripheral Language Disorders		
Dysarthria	difficulty in articulation	motor cortex, brainstem, connecting pathways, or cranial nerves
Dysphonia	difficulty in vocalization	motor cortex, brainstem, connecting pathways, cranial or spinal nerves
Production Aphasias		
Broca's	nonfluent language production normal comprehension	Broca's area, language dominant hemisphere
Dysgraphia	inability to produce written language	Dejerine's area, language dominant hemisphere
Dysprosody	disruption of normal tone and rhythm of speech	Broca's area, nondominant hemisphere
Echolalia	ability to repeat but not initiate speech	(?) Dejerine's area, language dominant hemisphere
Nominal Aphasia	inability to find names	(?) Wernicke's area
Nonpropositional Speech	production of jargon or automatic speech; swearing; singing	extensive involvement of language dominant hemisphere
Receptive Aphasias		
Wernicke's	fluent but often meaningless speech; inability to comprehend language	Wernicke's area, language dominant hemisphere
Dyslexia	inability to comprehend written language	Dejerine's and Wernicke's areas, language dominant hemisphere
Auditory Agnosia	inability to comprehend spoken language	Wernicke's area, language dominant hemisphere
Global Aphasia	inability to comprehend or produce language	extensive involvement of language dominant hemisphere

from improper control of the muscles of either respiration or the vocal cords.

Cortical communication disorders, or *aphasias*, can be divided into receptive and expressive types. These disorders may affect either hemisphere and thus produce disturbances predominantly in either language function or nonsyntactic communication. Within each general type of aphasia, a number of subdisturbances are possible.

Spatial Perception

Spatial perception involves organizing parts of the external world in relationship to each other, our bodies in relationship to the external world, and parts of our bodies in relationship to each other. The parietal association cortex of the right hemisphere appears to be the major center for these functions, but the frontal association cortex also is involved. As with communication, the parietal lobe may be of major importance for receiving and processing spatial information; the frontal lobe may be essential for formulating movements permitting exploration of the environment by the eyes and through "active touch" with the fingers. Considerable evidence exists that active body movement is essential to the normal development of all types of spatial perception.

Spatial organization of the external world permits intellectual processes such as the following:

1. Pattern discrimination (including figure-ground discrimination).
2. Pattern identification.
3. Determination of object constancy.
4. Determination of relative object location.
5. Mapping of external space.

Vision is clearly the most important sensory modality for spatial organization of the external world, but auditory, tactile, and proprioceptive sensation also can supply valuable clues. Exploratory eye movements and active touch with the fingers are both valuable for determining spatial organization of external objects. Either exploratory method provides superior perception to that which can be generated through passive presentation of the object. The superiority seems to be the result of the combined additional information provided by internal cortical feedback of efference and reference data concerning movements of the eyes or the hands.

Generation of body image relies strongly on exteroceptive and proprioceptive input. Body image involves concepts of location of body parts relative to the body center (eg, left, right, front, back) and relative to each other. Relative size of body parts also is part of body image. Identification of the location of the entire body or parts of the body in relation to their center of gravity (center of mass) is a subconscious component of body image. This identification is dependent on proprioceptive information from muscle, tendon, and joint receptors (and probably skin receptors in the hand). Evidence of identification of center of gravity and the changes of the body in relation to it are seen in postural adjustment movements.

Relationship of the body to the surrounding world probably is generated on the basis of both of the above concepts. Exploratory body movements into surrounding space are necessary to generate a normal concept of the body-world relationship. Identification of the spatial relationship between the body or its parts and the external world may be either subconscious or brought to the level of perception. Proprioceptive systems, particularly the vestibular system, are important in generating body-world spatial relationships, as is the visual system. Other teloreceptive systems also can play a part in generating this information. One of the primary perceptions arising from the body-world relationship is that of verticality. Equilibrium and righting responses demonstrate the presence and appropriate use of verticality information.

Many types of dysfunction may exist in the area of spatial perception. They may be based on inappropriate reception or processing of sensory information, abnormal movement patterns, or lack of congruence between bits of information that are normally supportive. Inability to adjust the body normally in relationship to gravity is a fairly common problem that may be evidence of either a distortion of body image or of a loss or conflict in the perception of verticality.

Another type of spatial organization dysfunction seen fairly commonly in therapy is sensory neglect. With this problem, the person behaves as though part of the body or part of external space, or both, does not exist. Symptoms of neglect include behaviors such as eating food from only one half of a plate, writing on only half of a piece of paper, drawing only one half of a circle when instructed to draw an entire circle, dressing only half of the body, and consistently losing one's balance toward the neglected side. Neglect can occur because a basic component of all logical processes in the cortex is completion or closure of incomplete data sets. Under normal circumstances, the development of both sequential and spatial logic is dependent on the existence of closure, because complete sensory information is rarely, if ever, available. The logical ability to reach closure apparently is so strong that it can overcome major defects in information availability.

Review Exercises

19-1. You are treating a patient who greets you by smiling broadly, shaking your hand in a normal fashion, and swearing at you. As you proceed with treatment your patient continues to swear, sometimes in a pleasant tone of voice and sometimes in a more angry tone of voice, particularly when he is required to do a difficult task. He never uses ordinary grammatical language. You find that you can give instructions best by demonstrating the desired activity rather than by describing it. Where in the cerebral hemispheres is (are) this patient's lesion(s) located? Would you anticipate that any other functions other than those described might be affected by the lesion(s)?

19-2. Refer to Patient #2 in the Appendix. This patient frequently demonstrates neglect of or inattention to her left arm. She cannot consistently point to it when asked where her arm is. She is aware of stimuli applied to her arm but is unable to localize them. Would you describe this as a sensory or a perceptual problem? Where would you expect a lesion to be which would cause this problem?

19-3. Refer to Patient #2 in the Appendix. On the basis of what you currently know about this patient what type of communication deficits might you expect her to demonstrate? Consider how this might affect the style of communication you use with this patient.

20

Central Nervous System Fluids and Metabolism

Fluid Compartments

There are four fluid compartments in the CNS: the vascular, the cerebrospinal fluid (CSF), the extracellular fluid, and the intracellular fluid. The volumes of these compartments are summarized in Table 20-1.

Within the skull, the fluid compartment volume must remain essentially constant at all times because any change in volume will cause a change in pressure on the neural tissue. A decrease in volume with a consequent reduction in pressure reduces the ability of the fluid compartments, particularly the CSF compartment, to protect the neural tissue from trauma. An increase in volume and pressure will result in compression and displacement of neural tissue, usually with resulting damage and loss of function. Since the vertebral

TABLE 20-1. Volumes of Fluid Compartments of the Central Nervous System

Compartment	Average Volume	Rate of Fluid Production or Entry
Vascular	800 ml	55 ml/min/100 gm tissue
Cerebrospinal Fluid		500-600 ml/day
Total	140 ml	(completely renewed every 5-7 hrs)
Ventricles	23 ml	
Extracellular Fluid		
Grey Matter	18 ml/100 gm tissue	
White Matter	13 ml/100 gm tissue	
Intracellular Fluid	40-50 ml/100 gm tissue (higher % H_2O in grey matter)	

canal is not as rigid, these concerns are not as great for the spinal cord; however, in cases of spinal trauma, tissue edema is a significant factor in the subsequent loss of tissue and function.

Anatomy of CNS Arteries

The arterial supply to the CNS has the primary characteristic of permitting overlapping supply from adjacent arteries. As a general rule, there is more than one route of supply for any given portion of the CNS. In reality, however, there are certain regions of the CNS for which the arterial supply is limited to the point of being easily compromised by trauma or disease. The basic pattern of arterial supply to the CNS is that of paired ventrally located arteries that send either penetrating or circumferential branch arteries into the substance of the nervous system (Fig. 20-1). The penetrating branches have radially organized zones that they supply; the circumferential branches supply regions that are organized longitudinally along the neuraxis. Typically, there are anastomoses between the ventral arteries, to the point in the adult of fusion of these arteries throughout most of the neuraxis. Overlap occurs regularly at the edges of radial zones and longitudinal regions of the penetrating and circumferential arteries.

The systemic arteries supplying the CNS are the carotid and vertebral arteries (Fig. 20-2). Small branches from the aorta provide additional supply to the spinal cord. The basic pattern of arterial supply is most nearly retained at maturity for the spinal cord (Fig. 20-3). The vertebral arteries in the lower medulla give rise to the paired ventral, or anterior, spinal arteries, which anastomose within one segment of their origin to form the midline anterior spinal artery. Circumferential branches of the vertebral arteries also give rise to the posterior spinal arteries, which remain separate the length of the spinal

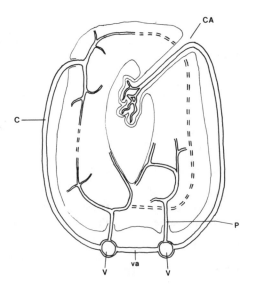

Figure 20-1. Basic pattern of CNS blood supply (cross-section of primitive neural tube). Paired ventral arteries *(V)* are connected by an anastomosis *(va)*. They project both circumferential *(C)* and penetrating *(P)* branches which will supply the CNS. Within the CNS smaller arterial branches occur along planes of dissection between major CNS regions; initially between the embryonic layers. Invaginating choroidal arteries *(CA)* arise from circumferential branches. Dorsal longitudinal branches (not shown) arise variably from circumferential branches in different regions of the CNS.

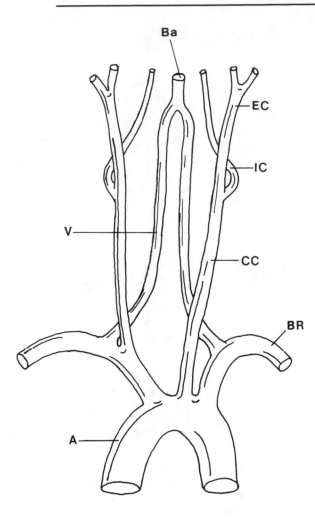

Ba

EC

IC

V

CC

BR

A

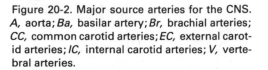

Figure 20-2. Major source arteries for the CNS. *A*, aorta; *Ba*, basilar artery; *Br*, brachial arteries; *CC*, common carotid arteries; *EC*, external carotid arteries; *IC*, internal carotid arteries; *V*, vertebral arteries.

cord. These longitudinal arteries are reinforced periodically by branches from segmental arteries. The arterial supply to the spinal cord is sufficiently redundant at most levels to overcome any limitations imposed by trauma. At the upper thoracic and lumbar levels, however, the ventral supply may easily be compromised, and the dorsal supply also is limited at the upper thoracic levels. These segments of the spinal cord therefore are prone to pathological condition as a result of vascular disorders or trauma affecting the vascular system.

The arterial supply pattern for the brainstem and cerebellum also is similar to the basic pattern. The main differences are the extensive rostral and caudal branching of the main circumferential arteries resulting from the enlargement of the cerebellum. From caudal to rostral the major circumferential arteries are the posterior inferior cerebellar, anterior inferior cerebellar, and superior cerebellar. These large circumferential arteries primarily supply the

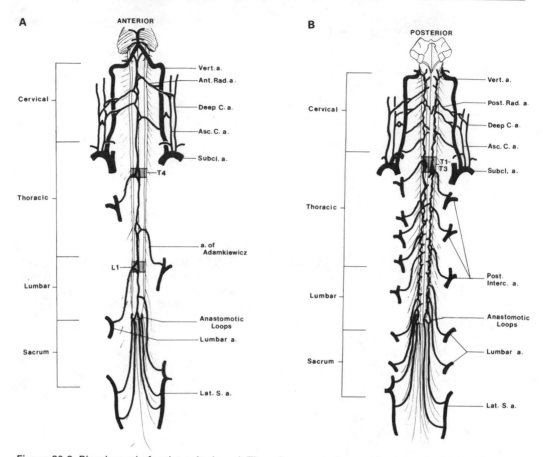

Figure 20-3. Blood supply for the spinal cord. The primary anterior supply shown in **A** arises from the vertebral arteries. Additional radicular supply arises from the descending aorta and its branches. The anterior spinal cord (ventral horn and adjacent tracts) has a limited arterial supply at the T-4 and L-1 levels. The posterior supply shown in **B** comes through paired posterior longitudinal arteries which arise from the vertebral arteries and from circumferential branches from radicular arteries and the single anterior spinal artery. The arterial supply to the dorsal horn and adjacent tracts is limited at levels T-1 through T-3. *Asc. C. a.,* ascending cervical artery; *Deep C. A.,* deep cervical artery; *Lat. S. a.,* lateral sacral artery; *Subcl. a.,* subclavian artery; *Vert. a.,* vertebral artery.

cerebellum, giving rise, in passing, to penetrating branches to the appropriate levels of the brainstem. For the most part, however, the brainstem is supplied by penetrating branches arising either directly from the basilar artery or from small circumferential arteries (Fig. 20-4). These penetrating branches supply three definite radial zones in the brainstem, with minimal overlap among zones. The penetrating branches typically arise from their parent arteries at nearly 90° angles. This abrupt change in direction of flow makes the origin of these arteries likely locations for arterial occlusion. As a result, the brainstem can develop small, petechial hemorrahages or regions of localized occlusion, resulting in very specific losses of function.

As a result of the immense enlargement and folding of the neuraxis at and

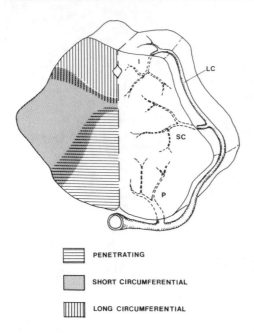

PENETRATING

SHORT CIRCUMFERENTIAL

LONG CIRCUMFERENTIAL

Figure 20-4. Basic pattern of arterial supply of the brainstem. The basilar artery gives rise to three sets of paired arteries: Penetrating arteries *(P)* arising from the basilar directly or from the proximal portion of the circumferential arteries; short circumferential arteries *(SC);* and long circumferential arteries *(LC)*. The cerebellar arteries are extended long circumferential arteries. Within the substance of the brainstem there is overlap between adjacent supply territories. Note the abrupt angle of departure of the penetrating arteries.

above the level of the diencephalon, the arterial supply to this region at maturity looks very different from the basic pattern. However, a primary, paired ventral supply with circumferential and penetrating branches can still be identified. The ventral arteries are the internal carotids with their anterior and posterior extensions (the anterior cerebral and the posterior communicating arteries) of each side. From caudal to rostral, the circumferential arteries are the posterior and the middle cerebral arteries. Ventrally, there is an anterior anastomosis between the anterior cerebral arteries, which is the anterior communicating artery. The basilar artery continues upward from the brainstem and divides to anastomose with both posterior communicating arteries, thereby forming the posterior cerebral arteries that complete the arterial anastomotic circle of Willis around the base of the brain (Fig. 20-5). The penetrating branches of greatest clinical importance are the anterior and posterior choroidal arteries, which supply the choroid plexus of the lateral and third ventricles, and the lenticulostriate penetrating branches of the anterior and middle cerebral arteries ,which supply the hemispheric basal ganglia and the internal capsule. The thalamus is supplied by the choroidal arteries and the penetrating branches from the posterior cerebral artery. The regions supplied by each major cerebral and diencephalic artery are diagrammed in Figures 20-6 and 20-7. The anterior cerebral artery is the major source of blood for the midline portion of the frontal lobe. The middle cerebral artery supplies the insula and the more lateral portions of the frontal lobe and most of the parietal and temporal lobes. The posterior cerebral artery supplies the occipital lobe and some of the parietal and temporal lobes. In the dorsum of each hemisphere, there is considerable overlap among the regions supplied by each artery.

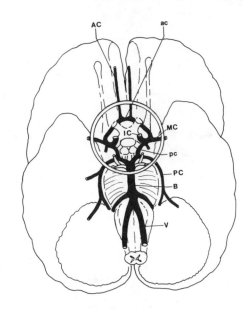

Figure 20-5. Components of the circle of Willis at the base of the cerebral hemispheres. *AC,* anterior cerebral artery; *ac,* anterior communicating artery; *B,* basilar artery; *IC,* internal carotid artery; *MC,* middle cerebral artery; *PC,* posterior cerebral artery; *pc,* posterior communicating artery.

Despite the ventral anastomoses of the circle of Willis and the overlap among supply regions of the circumferential arteries, the functional redundancy of blood supply to the cerebrum appears to be quite limited under normal circumstances. In cases of slowly developing arterial occlusion of the main arteries leading into the circle of Willis, functional anastomotic supply can develop to a certain extent. When loss of blood supply occurs rapidly, there is insufficient time for anastomotic flow to become functional and protect neural tissue from the effects of loss of blood flow.

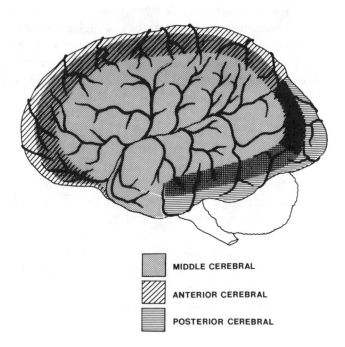

Figure 20-6. Arterial supply territories in the cerebral hemispheres, lateral view. The three major cerebral arteries (anterior, middle and posterior) each have unique territories with regions of potential overlap between adjacent territories. In the occipital lobe there is potential overlap in supply from all three arteries.

MIDDLE CEREBRAL

ANTERIOR CEREBRAL

POSTERIOR CEREBRAL

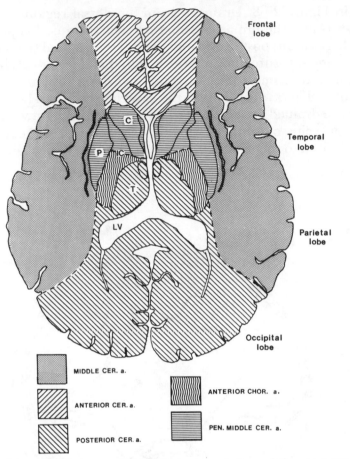

Figure 20-7. Arterial supply of the cerebral hemispheres and diencephalon, horizontal section. The anterior limb and part of the genu of the internal capsule is supplied via penetrating branches of the middle cerebral artery. The remainder of the internal capsule is supplied via branches of the anterior choroidal artery. *C*, caudate nucleus; *IC*, internal capsule; *LV*, lateral ventricle; *T*, thalamus; *P*, putamen.

Anatomy of CNS Veins

The venous system within the skull serves to receive fluid from the capillaries and the cerebrospinal fluid spaces. To a very limited extent, this system can serve the function of a volume-pressure buffer. Because of the normal location of the skull above the level of the heart, the larger cerebral veins are typically venous sinuses with considerable pressure capacitance and essentially no resistance to fluid flow. These sinuses do not collapse under conditions of low pressure or volume, because of the rigid surrounding structures of the skull and meninges. There are no valves within the cerebral venous system. Valves in the jugular veins just above or at the thoracic inlet are sufficient to protect the cerebral circulation from back-flow volume and pressure changes resulting from changes in intrathoracic pressure. Major intracranial veins are illustrated in Figure 20-8. Drainage from the dorsal regions of the cerebral hemispheres is into the unpaired superior sagittal sinus. Deeper portions of the hemispheres drain posteriorly into the inferior sagittal sinus located at the base of the sagittal fissure and anteriorly into the anterior cerebral vein. The diencephalon and its immediate surroundings drain primarily into the short great vein of Galen or directly into the cavernous sinus. The brainstem and cerebellum are drained by the petrosal sinuses and the great vein of Galen. All of these large veins or sinuses, with the exception of the cavernous sinus, eventually drain into the confluence of sinuses located midsagitally just above

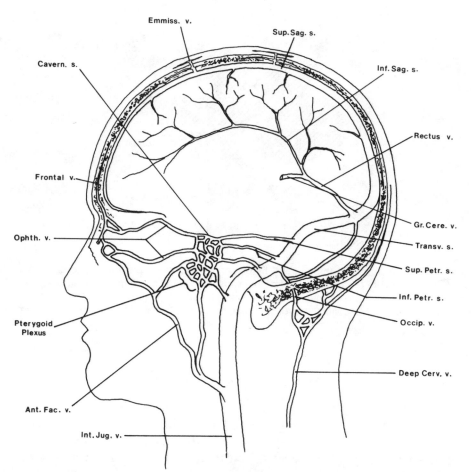

Figure 20-8. Major intracranial veins draining the central nervous system. The dorsal and superficial regions of the cerebral hemispheres drain into the superior sagittal sinus *(Sup. Sag. s.)*. Deeper regions of the hemispheres, the diencephalon, and the cerebellum drain into the inferior sagittal sinus *(Inf. Sag. s.)* located within the dura at the base of the falx cerebri and the great cerebral vein *(Gr. Cere. v.)* or vein of Galen. Structures at the base of the brain drain into the cavernous sinus *(Cavern. s.)*. The primary route of exit from the cranium is the paired internal jugular veins which collect blood from the cavernous and pterygoid sinuses and the paired transverse sinuses *(Transv. s.)*. The deep cervical vein provides a minor exit route. The small emmissary veins *(Emmiss. v.)* penetrating the cranial bone drain deep layers of this bone and can provide routes for transmission of superficial infections into the central nervous system.

the posterior limit of the tentorium, within the falx cerebri. From this juncture, the paired transverse sinuses carry the venous blood to the internal jugular veins. The cavernous sinus can empty partially into the petrosal sinuses. By way of the pterygoid venous plexus blood from the cavernous sinus eventually can join the internal jugular vein in the neck. Due to the multiple drainage routes available within the cerebral circulation and the rigid structure of the meninges surrounding the principal sinuses, occlusion of the cerebral venous system is rare.

Cerebral Blood Flow

The average cerebral blood flow is maintained at a value of 55 ml/min/100 gm tissue over a range of systemic blood pressures of 60 to 150 mmHg. A decrease in flow rate below this level would jeopardize metabolism. Any significant increase in flow rate would be likely to affect the physical properties of the capillaries and lead to cerebral edema as a result of bulk flow out of the capillaries. Short term control of cerebral blood flow rate appears to be predominantly autoregulatory. Metabolic factors implicated in cerebral autoregulation are similar to those in any other tissue: extracellular concentrations of potassium, lactate, carbon dioxide, and adenosine. Evidence for the importance of these factors comes from the rapid alterations in local cerebral flow in response to changes in neural activity. Alterations in arterial partial pressure of carbon dioxide (within normal limits) do not appear to have a direct effect on cerebral vascular smooth muscle.

Additionally, cerebral vessels have autonomic innervation. As in other parts of the circulation, sympathetic norepinephrine causes vasoconstriction. Parasympathetic innervation appears to be present in the cerebral circulation. Acetylcholine causes vasodilitation. There is uncertainty about the availability of receptors for circulating epinephrine. Although neurotransmitters potentially can bring about rapid changes in local or general cerebral blood flow, they appear to do so only in cases of pathological changes in flow. Under normal circumstances, the autonomic innervation of the cerebral circulation appears to be used to provide tonic input that may have as much a trophic as a direct excitatory or inhibitory effect on vascular smooth muscle. For example, prolonged elevation of sympathetic activity leads to a significant hypertrophy of cerebral vascular smooth muscle.

Cerebral vascular smooth muscle also responds reflexively to abrupt changes in perfusion pressure. An increase in pressure induces a brief vasodilitation followed by vasoconstriction that lasts for the duration of the pressure elevation. The opposite response is seen with a drop in perfusion pressure. These pressure reflex responses protect the brain from rapid alterations in blood supply and serve to maintain the intracranial volume at a constant value.

Circulation of Cerebrospinal Fluid

Entry of fluid into the CNS can occur by bulk flow at either the capillary-extracellular fluid interface or the capillary-cerebrospinal fluid interface in the choroid plexi of the ventricles. The net flow across the latter interface is by far the greater. Fluid is removed from the CNS primarily through the arachnoid villi of the cerebrospinal fluid system. Some fluid also reenters the vascular compartment through the capillaries (Fig. 20-9).

Solute concentrations differ significantly between the cerebral circulation and the cerebrospinal fluid, as indicated in Table 20-2. These differences are due to regulation of solute movement at the blood-extracellular fluid interface (blood-brain barrier) and the choroid plexi. Diffusion in both cases is governed as usual only by the diffusing capacity of the solutes through the membranes of the cells of the interface.

Movement of solutes requiring active or facilitated transport can be regulated. Movement of solutes across the blood-brain barrier is summarized in Table 20-3. Note that only oxygen and carbon dioxide diffuse freely at this interface. The apparent diffusion of carbon dioxide is actually a movement of hydrogen ions as a result of chemical interactions with bicarbonate in both fluid spaces.

Neurotransmitters are broken down by enzymes in the endothelial cells, blocking nonspecific release of active substances into the general circulation and nonspecific uptake of transmitters into the CNS. (Neurotransmitters are released nonspecifically by some neurons into the CSF and distributed by this route to appropriate target cells within the CNS).

At certain sites within the brain, the capillary endothelium is much more open, permitting free exchange of solutes through bulk flow. These regions

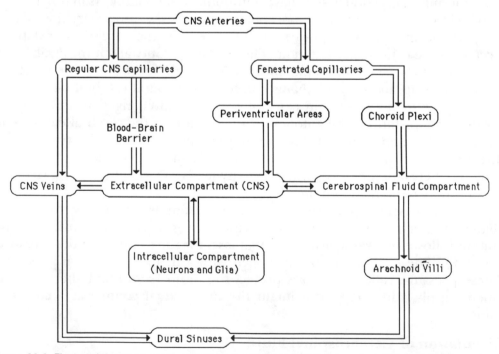

Figure 20-9. Flow pathways connecting fluid compartments within the central nervous system.

TABLE 20-2. Comparison of Solute Concentrations in Plasma and Cerebrospinal Fluid*

Solute	Plasma Concentration	CSF Concentration
Magnesium (mM)	4.63	2.86
Calcium (mM)	2.35	1.14
Bicarbonate (mM)	99.00	113.00
Inorganic phosphate (mg/100 cm^3)	26.8	23.3
Protein (mg/100 cm^3)	6800.00	28.00
Glucose (mg/100 cm^3)	110.00	50-80
P_{CO2} (mmHg)	41.10	50.50
pH	7.397	7.307

*Solutes not listed have concentration ratios very close to 1.0

appear to serve either the important sensory functions (eg, glucose concentration sampling by hypothalamic glucostats) or the release of neurohormones into the systemic circulation as occurs in the hypothalamic-pituitary system.

The choroid plexi are secretory epithelium (Fig. 20-10). In the choroid plexi, water enters the CSF down an osmotic pressure gradient produced by a net influx of sodium into the CSF at this site. Bulk flow of water and some solutes can occur also at "pores" in the choroid epithelium. Solute transport into the CSF is limited in ways similar to those seen at the blood-brain barrier. Some solutes existing in relatively high concentration in the CSF, such as amino acids and neurotransmitters, leave the CSF in the choroid plexi and either enter the circulation or are broken down by the capillary endothelium. The capillary endothelium in the choroid plexi is very open, permitting free exchange of water and solutes between the plasma and the extracellular fluid space. The epithelium is the location of the primary barrier to bulk flow and free exchange of water and solutes. The surface area at which the cerebrospinal fluid is produced is extensive as a result of both the convolutions of the plexi and the presence of microvilli on the ventricular side of the epithelial cells.

TABLE 20-3. Fluid and Solute Movement Across the Blood-Brain Barrier

Component	Diffusion	Facilitated Transport	Active Transport
H_2O	X	X	
O_2	X		
CO_2 (as H^+)	X		
Lipid-Soluble, Nonpolar Solutes (eg, ethanol, heroin)	X		
Glucose		X	
Ketones		X	
Lactate, Pyruvate		X	
Amino Acids		X	
Water-Soluble Vitamins (eg, ascorbate, folate, inisotol)			X
NOT Exchanged: · neurotransmitters · proteins · ions (net exchange = 0); except H^+			

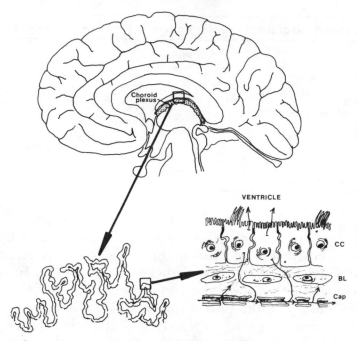

Figure 20-10. Location and structure of the choroid plexus. Choroid is found in the third ventricle (shown, top), the lateral ventricles and the fourth ventricle. The choroid epithelium forms a highly convoluted tissue providing a large secretory surface area (bottom left). This tissue is made up of a loosely organized basement layer *(BL)* and a secretory layer of cuboidal cells with microvilli *(CC)*. These cells permit secretory passage of fluids and solutes into the ventricles while blocking free exchange through desmosomes or tight junctions. The secretory epithelium is supplied with a network of fenestrated choroidal capillaries *(Cap.)*.

After production in the choroid plexi, the CSF circulates through the ventricles and enters the subarachnoid space through the foramina of Luschka and Magendie in the fourth ventricle. There is no barrier to exchange between the CSF and the neural extracellular fluid along the walls of the ventricular system. Once in the subarachnoid space, the CSF is barred from exchanging with the extracellular fluid of the CNS by the presence of the pia mater. All components of the CSF freely re-enter the vascular system through the arachnoid villi located in either the superior sagittal sinus or the radicular veins of the spinal cord (Fig. 20-11). Flow in these locations is the result of either bulk flow down a 4 to 5 mmHg pressure gradient or pinocytotic transport through the arachnoid cells in the villi.

Disruption of CSF Flow and Cerebral Edema

The most typical problems associated with CSF flow involve either excess production of CSF by the choroid plexi or occlusion of pathways, within the ventricular system or at the arachnoid villi. Problems related to insufficient CSF production are rare. Excess CSF production can result from tumors that cause malignant growth of the choroid tissue. Occlusion of flow within the ventricular system can result from either congenital malformations or pathological tissue shifts involving the narrow passageways connecting the ventricles or leaving the fourth ventricle. Blockage of sufficient arachnoid villi to cause cessation of CSF circulation occurs typically only as a result of infectious processes involving the brain or meninges. When excess CSF volume (hydro-

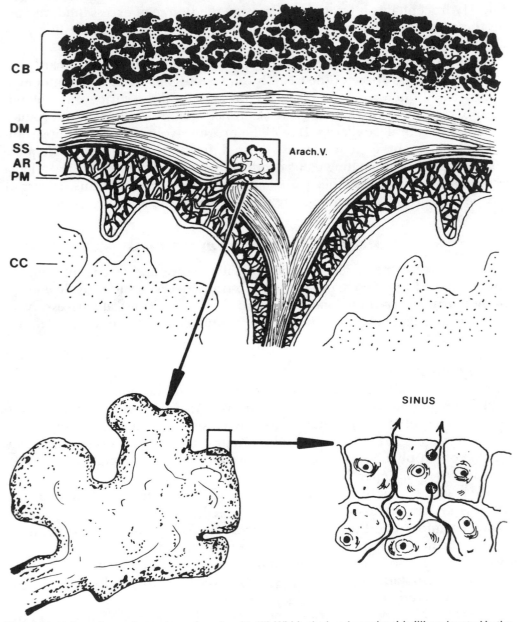

Figure 20-11. Location and structure of arachnoid villi. Within the head anachnoid villi are located in the superior saggital sinus (Top). They consist of a loosely packed and highly vascularized projection of the arachnoid into the sinus (bottom left). Fluid passage from the subarachnoid space through these villi and into the sinus can be effected either through movement between the surface cells down the small but consistent pressure gradient or through pinocytosis. Secretory processes are not involved. *AR,* arachnoid with trabeculae bridging the subarachnoid space; *CB,* cortical bone; *CC,* cerebral cortex; *DM,* dura mater; *PM,* pia mater.

cephalus) occurs congenitally, the skull can expand in response to the increased intracranial pressure. Damage to neural tissue thus is minimized. When hydrocephalus occurs after the sutures of the skull have closed, the result is an increase in pressure within the skull. Neural tissue is damaged as a result of shifts in tissue position and by pressure-induced occlusion of blood flow. Hydrocephalus is treated by removing the source of excess fluid, removing the cause of occlusion, or providing an alternative exit route (shunt) for the excess fluid.

Cerebral edema differs from hydrocephalus in that it involves primarily the extracellular fluid space of the CNS. It can result from a variety of pathological processes, but a common factor is a decrease in the security of the blood-brain barrier, with a resulting increase in net bulk flow of water and solutes out of the cerebral capillaries. Due to the pressure-volume relationships within the skull, cerebral edema can also cause shifts in tissue and loss of adequate blood supply, with resulting tissue death and loss of function. Cerebral edema secondary to trauma or other pathology is probably a greater cause of loss of function in the entire CNS than the primary pathology in many cases.

Metabolic Substrate For Neurons

The substrates necessary for normal maintenance and activity of neurons can be divided into two major classes: substrates necessary to provide energy, in the form of creatine phosphate and ATP, and substrate necessary to support anabolic functions, such as the manufacture of specific transmitter molecules.

Energy Substrate

For energy substrate, the brain, under normal conditions, relies almost entirely on glucose and oxygen to support oxidative phosphorylation. The use of substrates other than glucose for glycolysis is extremely limited; even alternate sugars are not used readily. Neural tissue is also only minimally capable of supplying its energy needs through anaerobic metabolism; therefore, it is oxygen dependent.

Given these basic conditions, it can be seen that the metabolism of the nervous system is relatively inflexible in quality under normal conditions. However, under conditions of sustained limited availability of glucose, as in fasting, the neurons can produce enzymes permitting the use of ketone bodies (two carbon products of fatty acid catalysis) as a substrate for the tricarboxylic acid cycle. This adaptive change is fully reversible when adequate glucose intake is restored.

The rate of glucose use varies depending on the type of CNS tissue and the amount of activity in that tissue. At rest, grey matter uses on the average 8.5 ml/100 gm tissue/min; white matter uses about half that amount. Active grey matter can increase its glucose use by at least a factor of 10. Under conditions of core body temperature lowering, the activity of neurons significantly decreases, raising the resistance of the CNS to anoxia. Changes necessary to support this wide range of metabolic rate include local changes in cerebral blood flow, general changes in mean cerebral perfusion (which nevertheless does not vary as greatly as the mean perfusion of some other tissues, such as muscle), and changes in arteriovenous oxygen difference. Changes in blood flow and oxygen extraction normally occur in parallel, but under some pathological conditions they may vary inversely or otherwise not show a normal response to anticipated increases in neural activity. For this reason, both blood flow changes and oxygen extraction should be evaluated when determining the metabolic capacity of a portion of the CNS.

Anabolic Substrate

The anabolic substrate for neurotransmitter synthesis can be determined from a review of the synthetic pathways. There are three basic categories: choline, precursor to acetylcholine; the amino acids tryptophan and tyrosine, precursors to serotonin and the monoamine transmitter group; and glucose, which acts as a precursor to a wide variety of peptide and amino acid transmitters through transamination of tricarboxylic acid cycle intermediates. Additional intermediate metabolites or final transmitters may be used directly by neurons, but their availability is severely limited by the permeability characteristics of the blood-brain barrier.

Central Nervous System Imaging Techniques

A number of techniques for visualizing the CNS have been developed in recent years. Many of these are based on known metabolic principles and are capable of providing physiologic as well as anatomic information about the system. The major imaging techniques used for the CNS, their general limitations and capabilities, and the theory on which they are based, are outlined below. Any one or a combination of these techniques are used for diagnostic purposes for various suspected CNS pathological states.

Imaging Techniques Based on Visualization of Structures

Classical Roentgenography. Use of variation in absorption of x-radiation by various tissues, to provide a static image of structures. This imaging technique can differentiate only between definitely radiopaque and radiolucent structures and therefore is not useful in imaging soft structures, such as brain tissue, in which there is a minimal range of radiodensity. Skull abnormalities and displacement of the midline pineal gland (usually calcified in adults) can be visualized very accurately with this technique.

Computerized Tomography (CT Scan). Use of precisely collimated ("focused") beams of x-rays collected by an array of scintillation crystals placed around the head in a single plane along a standard axis. Multiple radiation transits of a single layer of tissue are summed to permit differentiation of radiodensity among various CNS tissues. Usually, many "slices" are imaged along the standard axis. This technique permits structural imaging of CNS soft tissue with a maximum resolution in the range of one millimeter. It is useful for visualizing changes in size and position of major CNS structures and for identifying relatively minor changes in radiodensity of structures, both of which can reflect pathological changes in tissue. Radioenhancer chemicals may be introduced by way of the circulatory system prior to the CT scan, to permit clearer visualization of the tissues that take up the particular chemical used.

Pneumoencephalography. Replacement of small volume of cerebrospinal fluid with air, to increase the contrast between soft tissue and fluid spaces in the brain or spinal cord. This technique permits visualization of the CSF fluid spaces, and thus of the outline of CNS soft tissue. It is rarely used currently because of the associated pain and inherent risk. For the most part it has been replaced by CT scans or other imaging techniques.

Cerebral Arteriography. Injection of a radiopaque substance into the vascular system. This technique, at various times following injection, permits contrast visualization of major arteries, minor vessels, and veins of the CNS. It is useful for direct visualization of CNS vasculature, and it can indicate regions of abnormal (increased or decreased) blood flow and abnormalities in vascular structure. It can also provide an outline image of CNS soft tissue.

Visualization Techniques Based on Metabolic Activity

Positron Emission Tomography (PET Scan). Vascular injection of radioisotopes, with subsequent uptake by brain tissue. The decay of the isotopes produces gamma radiation (positrons). This radiation is recorded using "slice" scanning techniques similar to those use in CT scans. Various isotopes are used that permit imaging of different structures or events, depending on the typical distribution of the isotope or the substance to which it is attached in CNS tissue. For example:

1. H^3 is distributed in water and thus permits imaging of the fluid spaces and the vasculature, depending on its mode of entry and the time following entry.
2. ^{18}F can be attached to glucose, permitting visualization of the location and degree of glucose use in various collections of neurons.
3. ^{11}C can be attached to certain compounds that bind to specific neurotransmitters or their receptors, permitting visualization of specific transmitter units or pathways.

One of the major values of the PET scan procedure is that it permits visualization of function while it is occurring. The spatial resolution is still limited to about 2 to 8 mm, with the degree of resolution being dependent on the isotope used.

Magnetic Resonance Imaging (MRI or NMR). Observation of the resonance and relaxation time of specific nuclei in a strong magnetic field. This technique has numerous advantages: It is completely noninvasive, it has a resolution on the order of 1 mm or less (equivalent to fixed anatomical sections), and it can provide both static and functional information. For example, hydrogen ion resonance information can give precise differentiation among tissues with slightly different water content and arrangement, permitting precise anatomic visualization of soft tissue. Phosphorus imaging can display the absolute and relative concentrations of phosphate compounds in neurons, permitting an analysis of their functional status.

Cerebral Thermography. Recording by thermal sensors of the relative temperature of the underlying central neural tissue. Changes in metabolic rate and associated blood flow lead to small but clearly detectable changes in temperature, which can be recorded from scalp sensors. The resolution of this technique is low compared with other imaging techniques. However, thermography, like magnetic resonance imaging, is completely noninvasive, and it requires less complex equipment than MRI.

These imaging techniques based on recording of effects of metabolic activity are particularly useful not only for diagnostic purposes but as research tools permitting examination of the function of the CNS.

Review Exercises

20-1.   Design a non-invasive experiment which could be used to demonstrate the validity of the localization, diffuse, or cellular connection theories. Consider what type of sensory or motor activity you would study and what types of observational methods you might use.

20-2.   Refer to Patient #2 in the Appendix. Show on Figures 20-5, 20-6 and 20-7 the location of the thrombosis and the probable areas of necrosis. Check your earlier responses relevant to this patient to see if they correlate with the lesion you have described.

20-3.   Refer to Patient #3 in the Appendix. Relate the identified changes in CNS fluid pressures and tissue location to the identified changes in visuomotor function you have already analyzed. What disruption would you anticipate in cerebrospinal fluid flow patterns? Can you suggest a relationship between changes in cerebrospinal fluid flow and extracellular fluid volume?

20-4.   Explain why dopamine, the neutrotransmitter which is deficient in Parkinson's disease, cannot be replaced by oral, intramuscular or intravascular administration.

20-5.   Refer to Patient #2 and Patient #3 in the Appendix. Setting aside concerns for patient safety (which vary with the pathology present) what type(s) of imaging technique would you use to confirm the presence of structural changes underlying the observed alterations in function? Justify your selection on the basis of the type of information you would obtain.

20-6.   What type(s) of imaging technique would you choose to conduct an experimental study on normal individuals aimed at determining 1) the regions of the CNS involved in producing walking behavior and 2) the sequence in which they are activated?

20-7.   In segments T-1 through T-4 of the spinal cord the blood supply is easily disrupted by even limited trauma in the area. Discuss the possible effect of such a lesion at this level on autonomic control of the heart.

APPENDIX

The four patients briefly described are referred to in various review exercises through the book. Only basic information is given in the Appendix; additional information about each patient is described with the relevant review exercises. All the problems in which the patient is cited are listed.

Patient #1. Referred to in the following review exercises: 1-1, 2-2, 5-3.

F.R. is a 52 year old farmer who suffered a crush injury to his right forearm while trying to repair some heavy equipment. The principal site of injury is over the ulna 17-20 cm proximal to the wrist (just below the elbow). There was a fracture of the ulna accompanied by trauma to all the extensor muscles in the forearm and crushing of the ulnar nerve over a distance of 1 cm (19 cm proximal to the wrist). The area of trauma was cleaned and the ulnar fracture stabilized with a plate three hours following the injury. The ulnar nerve was repaired with a graft from the sural nerve. Due to the extensive tissue disruption the fracture could not be stabilized with a cast.

Nerve conduction velocity examination conducted immediately prior to surgical repair gave the following results:

Motor conduction:
- Normal distal latency following stimulation of the ulnar nerve at the wrist
- No EMG response in the hypothenar muscles following stimulation of the ulnar nerve in the axilla
- No stimulation was tried at the elbow

Sensory conduction:
- Normal latency to stimulation of the little finger with recording electrodes at the wrist
- No response recorded in the axilla
- No recording was tried at the elbow

Additionally, no voluntary movement was possible for the intrinsic hand muscles innervated by the ulnar nerve, and the ulnar side of the palm was anesthetic to all stimuli.

Patient #2. Referred to in the following review exercises: 1-1, 13-3, 13-7, 17-1, 17-6, 19-2, 19-3, 20-5.

M.J. is a 68 year old woman who suffered a stroke (cerebrovascular accident, CVA) as a result of a thrombosis lodged at the point where the right middle cerebral artery branches from the internal carotid artery. She was medically stable within 48 hours of the stroke. When she is seen the next morning for initial evaluation she is mildly confused and is apparently having difficulty in recognizing people. At this time she needs assistance with all mobility activities, including bed mobility. By the time of discharge to a long-term care facility 8 days after the stroke she has progressed to being able to manage some bed mobility independently, to performing standing bed to chair transfers with assistance, and to performing some self-care activities such as eating and grooming with minimal assistance.

Patient #3. Referred to in the following review exercises: 1-1, 16-1, 16-3, 17-1, 17-2, 20-3, 20-5.

E.G. is a 19 year old man who suffered a closed head injury as the result of an automobile accident. Upon admission he was in coma. His vital signs were:

- heart rate   125 bpm
- blood pressure   85/70 mm Hg
- respiratory rate   25 breaths per minute
- core temperature   97° F

Visualization of the CNS demonstrated the presence of a subdural hematoma over the left cerebral hemisphere. There was also evidence of cerebral edema. The left cerebral hemisphere was compressed and the medial portion of the temporal lobe was displaced downwards past the tentorial notch. The hematoma was surgically evacuated and bleeding stopped. The cerebral edema was managed with drug therapy.

E.G. remained in a coma for 16 days. Upon regaining consciousness he was confused and restless with periods of combativeness for the next 3 weeks. During rehabilitation E.G. showed significant functional recovery, but at discharge 3 months following the injury he still had both cognitive and motor functional deficits.

Patient #4. Referred to in the following review exercises: 1-1, 7-2, 13-6, 15-3, 16-2, 16-3, 16-4.

S.J. is a 24 year old man who suffered a fracture with anterior dislocation of vertebra C5 on C6. The dislocation was reduced immediately following admission and the cervical region was stabilized with halo traction for the following two months. Various evaluations suggested the following pattern of tissue disruption:

a. Interruption at the C6 level of the following tracts:
   left:
      all tracts in the dorsal, lateral and ventral funiculi
   right:
      dorsal columns
      lateral corticospinal tract
      dorsal spinocerebellar tract

lateral reticulospinal tract

dorsal portions of the lateral spinothalamic and anterior
   spinocerebellar tracts

portions of the propriospinal tracts adjacent to the dorsal horn

b. necrosis at the C5-C6 level of the following laminae

left:

all laminae

right:

laminae I-IV

lateral portion of lamina V

SUGGESTED READING

ATLASES

DeArmond SJ, Fusco MM, Dewey MM: Structure of the Human Brain. 3rd ed. New York, New York: *Oxford University Press*, 1989.

Haines DE: Neuroanatomy. An Atlas of Structures, Sections and Systems. 2nd ed. Baltimore, Maryland: *Urban & Schwarzburg*, 1987.

Roberts M, Hanaway J, Morest DK: Atlas of the Human Brain in Section. 2nd ed. Philadelphia, Pennsylvania: *Lea & Febiger*, 1987.

COMPLETE TEXTS

Carpenter MB, Sutin J: Human neuroanatomy. 8th ed. Baltimore, Maryland: *Williams and Wilkins*, 1983.

Kandel ER, Schwartz JH: Principles of Neural Science. 2nd ed. New York, New York, *Elsevier*, 1985.

Netter FH: Nervous system Part I: Anatomy and Physiology. The *Ciba* Collection of Medical Illustrations, Vol. I, *Ciba Pharmaceutical Co.*, 1983.

PHYSIOLOGY TEXTS WITH NEUROSCIENCE SECTIONS

Berne RM, Levy MN: Physiology. 2nd ed. St. Louis, Missouri: *C.V. Mosby*, 1988.

Guyton AC: Textbook of Medical Physiology. 7th ed. Philadelphia, Pennsylvania: *W.B. Saunders*, 1986.

SPECIALIZED TEXTS

Brooks VB: The Neural Basis of Motor Control. New York, New York: *Oxford University Press*, 1986.

Ito, M. The Cerebellum and Neural Control. New York, New York: *Raven Press*, 1984.

Lund JS, ed: Sensory Processing in the Mammalian Brain. Neural Substrates and Experimental Strategies. New York, New York: *Oxford University Press*, 1989.

Miller N: Dyspraxia and Its Management. Rockville, Maryland: *Aspen* 1986.

Peterson BW, Richmond FJ: Control of Head Movement. New York, New York: *Oxford University Press*, 1988.

Phillips CG: Movements of the Hand. The Sherrington Lectures XVII. Liverpool, England: *Liverpool University Press*, 1986.

Shepherd GM: The Synaptic Organization of the Brain. 2nd ed. New York, New York: *Oxford University Press*, 1979.

Willis WD. The Pain System. The Neural Basis of Nociceptive Transmission in the Mammalian Nervous system. New York, New York: *S. Karger*, 1985.

INDEX

Page numbers in **bold face** refer to illustrations.